HEALTH ANXIETY AND THE QUEST FOR SAFETY

Health Anxiety and the Quest for Safety critically examines how psychological and sociocultural processes influence anxiety and safety-seeking behaviour concerning perceived health risks in globalised information societies. It provides insights into how people respond to uncertainty and perceived threats to their body and health in the 'age of anxiety'.

In examining the history of health anxiety, the author explores fluctuations in concepts, highlighting the power dynamics, uncertainties, and biased social and scientific attitudes in the background. The chapters offer a critical analysis of contemporary safety-seeking strategies, including online health information searches, fad diets, self-tracking, body image interventions, and the pursuit of personal meaning and well-being. Additionally, the book investigates how sociocultural influences can induce guilt about one's body and health, promote self-blame, or foster stigmatising attitudes while emphasising how the emergence of 'psy-culture', pop psychology, and digital tools may not only enhance health empowerment but also generate health-related anxieties and deepen inequalities. As a critical reflection on prevailing individualistic paradigms, the work also considers concepts that emphasise resonance and connectedness.

This book is valuable reading for clinical and health psychologists, critical social scientists, researchers, and students in the health sciences, as well as practitioners in all healthcare settings, psychotherapists, and communication specialists.

Márta Csabai is a clinical and health psychologist and a full professor at the Institute of Psychology at Károli Gáspár University of the Reformed Church in Budapest, Hungary.

Critical Approaches to Health

Series Editors

Kerry Chamberlain & Antonia Lyons

The Routledge Critical Approaches to Health series aims to present critical, inter-disciplinary books around psychological, social and cultural issues related to health. Each volume in the series provides a critical approach to a particular issue or important topic, and is of interest and relevance to students and practitioners across the social sciences. The series is produced in association with the International Society of Critical Health Psychology (ISCHP).

Titles in the series:

Making Mental Health
A Global History
Elizabeth Roberts-Pedersen

Critical approaches to death, dying and bereavement
Erica Borgstrom and Renske Visser

Critical Health and Learning Disabilities
An Exploration of Erasure and Social Murder
Sara Ryan

Health Anxiety and the Quest for Safety
Interdisciplinary and Critical Perspectives
Márta Csabai

For more information about this series, please visit: https://www.routledge.com/Critical-Approaches-to-Health/book-series/CRITHEA

HEALTH ANXIETY AND THE QUEST FOR SAFETY

Interdisciplinary and Critical Perspectives

Márta Csabai

Routledge
Taylor & Francis Group
LONDON AND NEW YORK

Designed cover image: Getty Images

First published 2026
by Routledge
4 Park Square, Milton Park, Abingdon, Oxon OX14 4RN

and by Routledge
605 Third Avenue, New York, NY 10158

Routledge is an imprint of the Taylor & Francis Group, an informa business

British Library Cataloguing-in-Publication Data
A catalogue record for this book is available from the British Library

ISBN: 978-1-032-85358-1 (hbk)
ISBN: 978-1-032-85357-4 (pbk)
ISBN: 978-1-003-51778-8 (ebk)

DOI: 10.4324/9781003517788

The Open Access version of this book was funded by Knowledge Unlatched.

An electronic version of this book is freely available, thanks to the support of libraries working with Knowledge Unlatched (KU). KU is a collaborative initiative designed to make high quality books Open Access for the public good. The Open Access ISBN for this book is 9781003517788. More information about the initiative and links to the Open Access version can be found at www.knowledgeunlatched.org.

For Product Safety Concerns and Information please contact our EU representative GPSR@taylorandfrancis.com. Taylor & Francis Verlag GmbH, Kaufingerstraße 24, 80331 München, Germany.

CONTENTS

SERIES EDITOR PREFACE

Critical approaches to health

Health is a major issue for people all around the world and is fundamental to individual well-being, personal achievements, and satisfaction, as well as to families, communities, and societies. It is also embedded in social notions of participation and citizenship. Much has been written about health, from a variety of perspectives and disciplines, but a lot of this writing takes a biomedical and positivist approach to health matters, neglecting the historical, social, and cultural contexts and environments within which health is experienced, understood, and practised. We developed this series of books to offer critical social science perspectives on important, relevant, and timely health topics.

The Critical Approaches to Health series provides new writing on health by presenting books that offer critical, interdisciplinary, and theoretical writing about health, where matters of health are framed quite broadly. The series seeks to include books ranging across important health matters, including general health-related issues (such as gender and media), major social issues for health (such as medicalisation, obesity, and palliative care), particular health concerns (such as pain, doctor-patient interaction, health services, and health technologies), particular health problems (such as diabetes, autoimmune disease, and medically unexplained illness), or health for specific groups of people (such as the health of migrants, the homeless, and the aged), or combinations of these.

The series seeks above all to promote critical thought about health matters. By critical, we mean going beyond the critique of the topic and work in the field, to more general considerations of power and benefit, and, in particular, to addressing concerns about whose understandings and interests are upheld and whose are marginalised by the approaches, findings, and practices in these various domains of health. Such critical agendas involve reflections on what constitutes knowledge, how it is created, and how it is used. Accordingly, critical approaches consider epistemological and theoretical positioning, as well as issues of methodology and practice, and seek to examine how health is enmeshed within broader social relations and structures. Books within this series take up this challenge and seek to provide new insights and understandings by applying a critical agenda to their topics. Explore the previous books in the series at *https://www.routledge.com/Critical-Approaches-to-Health/book-series/CRITHEA*.

In this book, *Health Anxiety and the Quest for Safety: Interdisciplinary and Critical Perspectives*, Márta Csabai brings together and critically considers a wide range of research and evidence from different fields with different terminologies, methodologies, and starting points. She provides valuable historical context, deftly orienting the reader to how work on anxiety and health has developed and how major events, including the COVID-19 pandemic, have altered both people's experiences and more general social understandings of what health anxiety is and how it plays an increasing part in our everyday lives.

From the outset, anxiety is framed as much more than an individualistic mental health issue, with Csabai taking a critical multidimensional approach and strongly arguing for consideration of different forms, including existential, ecological, and civilisational anxiety. Late modernity is seen as an 'age of anxiety' which has intensified with health threats arising through increasing globalisation and digitalisation of life. Csabai comprehensively pulls together scholarship from psychology, sociology, critical social theory, and cultural studies to show how perceptions, emotions, knowledge, social contexts, communication, and media all shape how we understand and experience health, risk, and anxiety. She draws on Beck's notion of a 'risk society' to consider how anxiety varies across historical contexts and generational cohorts facing specific societal challenges. She also critiques the medicalisation of health anxiety, giving attention to both old terms (e.g. hypochondria) and more recent ones (e.g. illness anxiety disorder, somatic symptom disorder, cyberchondria), to consider how they function in today's world.

These critical understandings of health anxiety are then applied to a range of different areas. The pervasive role of the internet in shaping and responding to anxiety is given particular attention, covering digital self-tracking methods and wearable technology, particularly in relation to stress management and relaxation, and how this feeds into self-management and understandings of health and well-being. Importantly, Csabai highlights how some of these digital tools reproduce inequalities. She reviews evidence on food, diet, and anxiety, including the contemporary obsession with healthy eating. This discussion is situated within broader cultural and environmental factors to do with the meanings of food, food production, and global food industries. Responsibility, blame, and guilt in relation to illness are also critically considered, as is research on body image and work on body-neutral and body-positive movements.

In the final chapter, Csabai broadens the focus and brings it back to people and well-being. She reviews research on how people find meaning and safety in a world that is challenging, complex, and frequently uncertain and argues for a holistic understanding of well-being that incorporates social, economic, and political systems. The book ends with clear directions for future scholarship that develops ways to promote and develop safer contexts that can reduce health anxiety in equitable and just ways.

This book takes up an important topic, considers it from a variety of positions and contexts, and draws together a wealth of research and theory that provides a substantial contribution to health anxiety scholarship, making a valuable addition to the Critical Approaches to Health series.

Antonia Lyons and Kerry Chamberlain
July 2025

1

ANXIETY IN A MULTIDIMENSIONAL FRAMEWORK

There is an increasing discussion in both academic and popular circles about anxiety as a symptom of modern society, which is considered particularly prevalent today as we are continuously confronted with potential threats from the world via the internet: news of epidemics, environmental disasters, wars, and technological hazards (Ackerley, 2024; Paulsen, 2024). This is supported by statistics from various countries, indicating that anxiety symptoms represent a significant proportion of mental health complaints (Schnittker, 2021). Considerable societal changes that heighten general uncertainties and threats to health and safety may further contribute to this trend. For instance, a global rise in anxiety complaints was noted during the COVID-19 pandemic, when concerns about health and safety surged among the general population and affected patients (Delpino et al., 2022; Pashazadeh et al., 2021). This issue continues to burden national health systems considerably (Javaid et al., 2023). In the United States, for instance, one-third of healthcare costs are spent on treating anxiety-related conditions (Single Care Team, 2022). However, the diversity and sometimes contradictory nature of social science and medical literature on anxiety raise important questions about how to interpret statistical data. One such question is whether anxiety can be regarded as an objective, quantifiable, and universally understood phenomenon (Malla & Gold, 2024). Additionally, it is essential to distinguish between adaptive forms of anxiety, which help individuals perceive and cope with real threats, and anxiety that impairs behaviour or may be classified as a mental disorder. Particularly relevant to this discussion is that contemporary anxieties frequently focus on health and bodily safety issues. These concerns deeply influence attitudes towards the body, risk perception, and health behaviours, all of which are significantly shaped by complex sociocultural factors. To further complicate the picture, social media and self-help pop psychology books present an idealised and simplistic view of anxiety-free living, contributing to the

DOI: 10.4324/9781003517788-1

rise of health anxiety as a rebound effect. All of these call for a critical and detailed approach.

The changing character of anxiety

A key factor in the development of health-related worries today is the invisibility and intangibility of anxiety-provoking elements, which may encompass elusive genetic differences as well as global environmental threats. In addition, the increased visibility of bodies on social media, along with messages that emphasise individual control over health and well-being – often in an unrealistic way – also plays a significant role in shaping health anxiety. While the sociocultural and political contexts of anxiety hold great significance, psychology, behavioural science, and psychiatry frequently concentrate excessively on individual experiences (Nightingale & Cromby, 2001). There is less consideration of the historical and sociocultural factors that have always shaped anxiety, perceptions of the body, health concerns, and risk assessment. With globalisation and the rise of mass societies, adopting a broader, multidisciplinary, and critical perspective has become crucial. This is particularly important, given the widespread notion that we live in an 'age of anxiety'. This concept has been discussed consistently in the social sciences since the mid-20th century (Smith, 2012a). Some researchers contend that each generation has experienced higher levels of anxiety during the 1900s than in those that preceded it (Stossel, 2014). However, others argue that this does not indicate an actual increase in clinically relevant anxiety cases but rather signifies a heightened public awareness of distress, which has brought about changed perceptions and concerns (Baxter et al., 2014). It is important to note that the mid-20th century coincided with the development of psychometric tools, which enabled the quantification of anxiety, even though the definition of anxiety itself is often unclear and varies.

Anxiety cannot be reduced to a one-dimensional phenomenon, making the definition of its clinical forms, like those of other mental health issues, a significant challenge. These categories are constructs shaped by ever-evolving scientific evidence and various theoretical perspectives. For instance, the *International Classification of Diseases* (ICD) and the *Diagnostic and Statistical Manual of Mental Disorders* (DSM) do not offer identical descriptions of anxiety (Schnittker, 2021). The DSM emphasises excessive worry and typically focuses on its chronic form, while the ICD highlights the acute form of anxiety. The ICD incorporates the classic concept of 'free-floating anxiety', which the DSM does not include. However, the DSM views anxiety as a cross-cutting phenomenon. Despite these differences in description, both systems define the prevalence of anxiety similarly. Additionally, the underlying psychological phenomena associated with anxiety are not inherently binary and cannot simply be categorised within the traditional medical model of normal versus abnormal functioning (Lahey et al., 2022). Critics have long argued that mental health phenomena resist strict categorisation and can be better understood as dimensions on a continuum (Widiger & Samuel, 2005). This may be one reason why international classifications of mental disorders are continually being updated and refined (Bandelow, 2017).

Today, a crucial factor in the development and characteristics of individual anxiety is the representation of scientific information about its prevalence in our societies as a mere fact, significantly shaped by the media and the internet. This information becomes incorporated into public perception, subsequently influencing behaviours and the formation of symptoms. According to the theory of social representation, this process creates a feedback loop that impacts the development of scientific theories, further reinforcing the social cycle of anxiety (Wagner, 2020). Social constructionist literature, particularly from the 1990s, argues that dominant cultural institutions shape the norms governing emotional production and expression (Heelas, 1998; Kitayama & Markus, 1994). They assert that anxiety as an emotion exists solely within a discursive framework; it can be identified only if it aligns with the labels and constructions prevalent in a particular social environment.

Adaptive and harmful anxiety

The above highlights the dilemma in psychological sciences regarding whether anxiety, primarily linked to the body, health, and existential security, can be more effectively understood through social constructionist and critical approaches situated within their cultural, political, and historical contexts. In contrast, conventional methods based on personality dimensions and psychopathology might explain anxiety more effectively in terms of the number of individuals diagnosed within specific groups or subgroups. Considering both approaches and their contributions to our understanding of anxiety would be valuable. Many professionals are questioning whether it is justified to unilaterally medicalise anxiety and treat it as a disease, which is also a feature of science, healthcare, and thus public thinking (Beeker et al., 2021; Frances, 2013). In recent decades, several studies have noted that concepts of harm – such as anxiety, depression, panic, trauma, and abuse – have become broader and more common. However, thls trend has not led to normalisation (Xiao et al., 2023). As discussed later in this volume, there has been an increase in pathologising discourses within both academic and public discussions. Numerous analyses have examined the potential adverse effects of medicalisation, a concern that is increasingly evident even in mainstream media coverage (Massey, 2019). Critical examinations highlight the dangers of labelling and stigmatisation (Fawcett et al., 2020). They also emphasise that the belief in the infallibility of medical solutions can lead to unrealistic expectations for external help, ultimately undermining the coping skills of those affected.

Even if we consider anxiety as a continuous spectrum rather than a simple binary construct, the question arises as to whether we can define an adaptive measure of anxiety, and when it becomes a problem that needs treatment. This task is complicated by the fact that anxiety can manifest in various emotional, behavioural, and physical forms and often does so indirectly – sometimes in ways that the individual might not even recognise. The challenge is further intensified by the strong subjective element inherent in anxiety, which is linked to a broad range of physical and mental health conditions. Consequently, it is difficult to measure and clearly distinguish what can be classified as 'natural' or 'normal' anxiety. For instance, the heightened anxiety experienced in the weeks following the attacks on the World Trade Centre on 11 September 2001 could be viewed as a natural response. However, the significant increase in the prescription of anti-anxiety medications in the United States immediately after this tragic event suggests a potential medicalisation of the issue. In New York alone, prescriptions rose by 22% (Druss & Marcus, 2004). During the 2008 economic crisis, there was also a notable increase in medication use (Stossel, 2014). Similarly, according to a scientific brief released by the World Health Organization (WHO), the COVID-19 pandemic resulted in a global rise of 25% in reported anxiety, with an estimated 76 million new registered cases in the first year (Brunier & Drysdale, 2022). This increased the average incidence rate from approximately 4,108.2 cases per 100,000 population to 5,588.6 (Santomauro et al., 2021). In India, for instance, 28% of the population experienced moderate to severe anxiety during the pandemic. In China, the figures were higher, with 33% overall and 38% among young people under 35 (Huang & Zhao, 2021). Interestingly, surveys from India revealed that one in four respondents began taking over-the-counter medications for anxiety during the COVID-19 pandemic, yet only 60% of these individuals fell into the high anxiety group (Chopra & Dasgupta, 2021). Given these statistics, the issue of interpretation and generalisability arises, considering the diversity of social and cultural representations of anxiety as reflected in the underlying data.

The experience of anxiety and its perception as a condition that requires treatment are shaped by various factors. Anti-anxiety medications may initially reduce anxiety, which encourages more medication use, but can also lead to increased anxiety over time due to this feedback loop (Tone, 2017). A notable example is panic disorder, which was the first psychiatric condition identified based on a specific drug mechanism in 1980. New York psychiatrist Donald Klein demonstrated that imipramine, a drug primarily used to treat depression, was also effective in relieving anxiety associated with panic (Stossel, 2014). As a result of various factors, panic disorder has emerged as one of the leading psychiatric conditions. This rise can be attributed, in part, to the availability of medications designed to treat it, along with the influence of pharmaceutical advertising and social media promotion. Patients often report symptoms of panic disorder to their doctors because they believe that the healthcare provider takes 'simple' anxiety and stress less seriously (Schnittker, 2021). Conversely, the use of psychiatric labels has become common for describing various feelings of discomfort (Xiao et al., 2023). The uncertainty surrounding the nature of the problem and the significant influence of socio-historical context are highlighted by the varying ways in which panic is experienced and understood across different cultures. For example, earlier cross-cultural studies have demonstrated that Americans arriving at emergency departments with panic-like symptoms typically feared a heart attack. In contrast, patients in Japan were more likely to be concerned about fainting (Lewis-Fernández & Kleinman, 1994).

An important question to consider is when an individual believes that a certain level of anxiety may be harmful to their health and when they should be concerned about it. A certain amount of worry is a natural part of our daily lives and can even be necessary for effective functioning. Charles Darwin (1872/1998), who suffered from agoraphobia – the fear of open spaces – experienced his condition to such an extent that he did not leave his house for years after his expedition on the Beagle (Kohn, 1963). Despite this, he noted that the 'capacity for fear' can enhance one's chances of survival, making it evolutionarily beneficial. Early 20th-century evolutionist authors argued that fear is advantageous, as it promotes safer behaviour, thus aiding the progress of civilisation (Adams, 1935). The philosopher Søren Kierkegaard argued that fear is essential for spiritual growth, stating, 'Whoever is educated by anxiety is educated by possibility' (Kierkegaard, 1844/2015, p. 156). The idea that anxiety impacts performance was emphasised in the early 20th century, especially during the first surge of psychological research (Yerkes & Dodson, 1908).

Following the Second World War, humanistic and existential psychologists argued that anxiety is vital for healthy development and is shaped by individual circumstances and sociocultural conditions (Kőváry, 2024). Rollo May, the leading figure in existential psychology, wrote in the preface to his book *The Meaning of Anxiety*:

> We are no longer prey to tigers and mastodons, but to damage to our self-esteem, ostracism by our group, or the threat of losing out in the competitive struggle. The form of fear has changed, but the experience remains relatively the same.
>
> *(May, 1977/2015, p. 3.)*

May attributed the rise in anxiety following the Second World War to various factors, including radical political movements, the looming threat of ongoing warfare, and the presence of the atomic bomb. Additionally, he highlighted individual issues, including inner confusion, uncertainty about personal values, and disorientation. By the 1970s, anxiety had gained such prominence that it became a marketable commodity, extending beyond the strict boundaries of scientific research (Stossel, 2014; Twenge, 2000). Interest in the subject surged significantly, especially considering that anxiety had only emerged as a distinct therapeutic field at the beginning of the 20th century. While people had experienced anxiety long before this, it was not typically regarded as a condition needing treatment, possibly due to the lack of therapeutic solutions available at the time. Thus, support and coping mechanisms were predominantly sought within the contexts of community and religion (Bourke, 2005). It was only after Sigmund Freud's work that anxiety began to be understood as a treatable psychological, neurophysiological, and psychosomatic issue (Freud, 1909/1990). Freud emphasised that addressing anxiety serves multiple purposes: it helps protect the self and plays a role in the development and maturation of the self. Thus, Freudian theory also suggests that anxiety has an adaptive function in an individual's life, aiding not just in the recognition and avoidance of danger but also in personality development. This notion is supported by subsequent psychological theories suggesting that effectively managing stress and overcoming anxiety associated with crises contribute to the maturation of personality (Erikson, 1956; Frankl, 1988). Nevertheless, the question remains whether we can ascertain the adaptive level of anxiety and to what extent individual characteristics versus other factors influence the increase in anxiety.

Civilised but anxious: the cost of progress?

Throughout the history of anxiety as a health issue, macro-level influences have received relatively less attention compared to individual processes. It is interesting to note, however, that even before Freud, a young New York physician named George Miller Beard explicitly linked the condition of neurasthenia to the development of civilisation in his semi-popular work, *American Nervousness* (Beard, 1881). He believed that ancient cultures could not have experienced nervousness due to the absence of steam power, the printing press, the telegraph, and a systematic scientific approach. In a misogynistic view, he also suggested that the ancient Greeks might have been more relaxed because women's intellectual contributions had not yet been recognised. Nevertheless, Beard's approach to understanding anxiety and functional symptoms was complex and well ahead of his time. Although he was a neurologist, he also considered the impact of social and lifestyle issues, such as the effects of overwork and excessive worry. Freud (1930/2002), partly influenced by Beard (1881) and acknowledging the complex nature of anxiety – both adaptive and harmful – argued in *Civilisation and Its Discontents* that all humanity could become neurotic under the pressures of civilising trends. He also drew heavily from the work of the French sociologist Émile Durkheim (1895/1982), who contended that the more we pursue pleasure, the more pain we expose ourselves to.

In the 20th century, with the rise of consumer society, the frustration of living better yet not necessarily being happier has intensified (Kahneman & Deaton, 2010). Since the latter half of the 20th century, more authors have suggested that modernisation has created conditions where we frequently feel stateless and alienated (Kőváry, 2024). Starting from the 1950s, the theme of anxiety became increasingly prominent in popular media and public discourse. Neurosis and nervous breakdowns became 'fashionable', often accompanied by physical symptoms, fatigue, somatic issues, and mild depression. This was also the period when anxiety medications, such as Valium, entered the mass market (Schnittker, 2021; Tone, 2017). Paradoxically, the rise in anxiety was fuelled by the expansion of psychotherapeutic culture (Stossel, 2014). As negative emotions shifted from the domain of religion to the realm of therapy, they became more individualised, contributing to a concurrent increase in anxiety (Bourke, 2005). Whereas these problems were previously regarded as influenced by transcendent and irrational factors beyond the individual's control, the focus has shifted to the individual, intensifying both personal responsibility and freedom of choice, thereby increasing anxiety. Since the mid-20th century, anxiety has come to signify not just illness but also a connection with busyness, performance, overwork, and stress (May, 1977). It appears to embody an inherent human condition in the fast-paced environment of mass society.

One of the key features of the 'postmodern condition' is the widespread anxiety among people concerning the loss of security and uncertainties about trust in knowledge and institutions (Bauman, 1998). This anxiety stems from the absence of singular, absolute principles that could provide a clear understanding of the world; instead, the world is now perceived as ambiguous, heterogeneous, and self-contradictory. In recent years, numerous studies on the culture of fear have emerged in academia and popular literature (Furedi, 2007). This concept dates to 1948 when the American poet W.H. Auden was awarded the Pulitzer Prize for his poem, *The Age of Anxiety*, in which he explored themes of identity and the fears of a man who has experienced war and the challenges of capitalism (Auden, 1947). Since the 1990s, there has been a notable increase in books that reference or are subtitled with the term 'age of anxiety' (Smith, 2012a, 2012b). Numerous publications with such titles have been released across various fields, including critical social history, art history, and fiction (Kholeif, 2021; Tone, 2017; Townshed, 2019). It has become a common sociological observation that society is marked by significant uncertainty and elevated levels of anxiety (Furedi, 2007). This phenomenon suggests that our understanding of the world is in a state of constant flux, neither stable nor predetermined.

During the significant social upheavals at the turn of the 20th century, as modernity began to take shape, there was widespread anxiety about changes to traditional social structures. In contrast, today's globalised, consumer-driven world offers us a seemingly endless array of choices in nearly every aspect of life. However, we often find these choices illusory; much of what is attractively advertised in the media is accessible only to a few people. The overwhelming stimulation and frustration from excessive choices often lead individuals into what is known as an existential vacuum (Frankl, 1988). Many attempt to avoid this vacuum by overworking, engaging in numerous activities, and constantly seeking to affirm their importance. This behaviour is partly driven by the fear that slowing down will confront them with a daunting sense of emptiness, which can evoke thoughts of ultimate meaninglessness. Interpreting the original concept of Frankl (1988) somewhat more narrowly, in contemporary society, this phenomenon is often referred to as the 'fear of missing out' (FOMO), which is particularly prevalent among younger generations and has been associated with various modern digital addictions and health anxieties (Elhai et al., 2021; Fitzgerald et al., 2022). Uncertainties and concerns regarding actual or perceived environmental threats complicate this further.

Intolerance of uncertainty and modern health worries

Zygmunt Bauman (2006) identifies vague, scattered, and unmoored anxieties as the predominant form of anxiety in our era, suggesting that attitudes towards uncertainty are influenced by how society perceives the relationship between the present and the future. Uncertainty will be felt more acutely and negatively if the future is perceived as more dangerous. Interestingly, particularly in Western societies, those who are often better off express more significant concerns about their safety and health, perhaps partly because they have more opportunities for self-expression and voicing their worries.

The issue of coping with and accepting uncertainty has recently gained attention in psychology, mainly through research on intolerance of uncertainty (McEvoy et al., 2019). A key finding in this area is the significant relationship of intolerance of uncertainty with health anxiety (Mazidi et al., 2024). Health-related intolerance of uncertainty is a key mediator between general intolerance of uncertainty and health anxiety, more so than worry, which is a secondary mediator. During COVID-19, intolerance of uncertainty also mediated between health anxiety and stress (Sorid et al., 2023). Worry influenced the link between intolerance of uncertainty and coronavirus anxiety; those with high trait worry and intolerance experienced the most COVID anxiety. These factors acted both independently and together as vulnerabilities to adverse psychological reactions to COVID-19. Interestingly, individuals treated for anxiety before the pandemic did not show any increased anxiety during COVID-19, unlike the general population (Rosmarin & Pirutinsky, 2024). This resilience is linked to the therapeutic tools that patients used to help them manage uncertainty. The authors state that anxiety results from intolerance of uncertainty, not uncertainty itself. This topic has recently gained media attention, such as of *The Guardian*, which emphasised that '[h]ealth anxiety can take over. Embracing uncertainty is crucial' (Straker & Winship, 2023). Some writings suggest strategies for overcoming intolerance of uncertainty and health anxiety, including recognising the positives of uncertainty, like interest, variety, and joy from surprises (Chesworth, 2022). A critical question is whether public discourse helps cope with uncertainty and anxiety or worsens it by emphasising these feelings.

Intolerance of uncertainty is strongly linked to 'modern health worries' (MHW) (Petrie et al., 2001), which are anxieties related to new environmental and technological issues. These worries stem from feeling uninformed and lacking control, especially when information is contradictory. Two types are identified: one relates to unknown, scientifically unobservable phenomena, and the other to perceived effects of uncontrollable, potentially catastrophic events that increase risk perception (Dömötör et al., 2019). The first scientific reports on MHW in the 2000s identified four primary areas of health concern: environmental pollution, toxic interventions, contaminated food, and radiation (Petrie et al., 2001). These concerns were significantly associated with somatic symptoms and the perceived value of health to individuals. Additionally, individuals with health anxiety tended to utilise healthcare services more frequently, especially alternative medicine. It is essential to recognise that this finding primarily pertains to Western societies and cannot be generalised globally. The authors suggest that MHW is influenced by popular media, which consistently highlights the potential 'dangers' to health, ranging from genetically modified foods to mobile phones and microplastics. The media tends to focus more on these external threats rather than on individuals' health behaviours, often fostering a sense of victimhood and vulnerability. Perhaps that's because the media are endeavouring to hold harmful commodity industries to account – including those companies and industries that pollute our water and soil in pursuit of profit.

MHW may also contribute to the persistence of medically unexplained symptoms despite ongoing improvements in diagnostic procedures (Jadhakhan et al., 2022). Cultural factors also play a significant role in shaping MHW. For instance, a study found that Swedes are particularly concerned about food safety, whereas New Zealanders worry more about environmental pollution's health effects (Palmquist et al., 2017). Another important aspect of MHW is that they are not closely linked to gender, age, education, personality traits, or specific disease constructs (Köteles et al., 2023). The connections to socio-economic status are less well understood; however, it has been found that individuals with higher levels of spirituality are particularly susceptible to overgeneralised messages regarding health-related risks (Köteles et al., 2016). As a result, individuals facing MHW often possess a more favourable attitude towards alternative medicine, astrology, and a holistic approach to health. Their perception of health risks may significantly influence their utilisation of health services, leading them to prioritise alternative forms of healing.

Perceiving risk: the power of communication

Risk perception is increasingly becoming a significant source of health anxiety today, as media and public discussions bring various dangers and their vaguely defined consequences to the forefront. One way to reduce anxiety is to understand the nature, type, and extent of potential hazards. However, this presents us with complex challenges, and we often struggle with even the most straightforward steps. According to Gerd Gigerenzer (2014), a leading international expert in risk theory and communication, one-third of the 1,000 people surveyed did not know the correct answer to the question of what 40% means. Specifically, they were asked which answers were correct: (a) 1 in 4, (b) 4 in 10, or (c) 1 in 40. As we will see in more examples below, one reason for this confusion may be that several psychological and sociocultural factors influence people's risk estimates beyond mathematical knowledge or skill.

The concept of risk today is more commonly associated with the fear of danger and harm, as well as concerns about the loss of health and security. Terms such as danger, threat, and disaster are increasingly linked to the concept of risk in both public discourse and the media (Lupton, 2023). This shift may stem from the growing importance of health and safety issues, as well as a lack of adequate policies and guidance for managing uncertainty, leading to a more negative perception of risk. This is reinforced by the fact that in neoliberal societies, individuals now must manage risks responsibly as part of their self-regulation (Crawford, 1980). There is a growing consensus that risk should be 'minimised', 'reduced', or 'avoided'. While extensive discussion exists about reducing risk, a key question remains: how quantifiable and measurable are risks and the associated anxieties? Another significant question, particularly from a critical standpoint, is why the quantitative approach is essential and whose interests it serves.

Several definitions of risk have emerged in recent decades, with two primary approaches becoming prominent. The first is the technical-scientific approach, which focuses on risk's measurable and objective aspects (Berry, 2004). The second is the sociocultural approach, which explores risk perception's social context and significance, allowing for symbolic interpretations. Both approaches acknowledge that zero risk – complete safety – is unattainable; there is always some level of risk involved in any action we take. A new critical approach in health risk research has developed in the past decade: *intersectionality*. This perspective emphasises the complex integration of traditional mathematical analyses with sociocultural viewpoints (Giritli-Nygren & Olofsson, 2014). Another psychological framework originates from the work of Black feminist scholar-activists and emphasises the interconnected systems of oppression, as well as the necessity of advocating for structural changes to improve social justice and equity (Rosenthal, 2016). Consequently, the increasing interest in intersectionality within psychology provides an opportunity for professionals to shift their focus towards structural issues, prioritising social justice and equity more prominently. The substantial and expanding body of research demonstrating the extensive detrimental effects of structural and interpersonal oppression, inequality, and stigma on the health and well-being of diverse communities underscores the necessity of addressing these issues in health risk studies as well.

In the past, decision theory primarily focused on rational, 'cold' processes. However, contemporary research on risk behaviour also incorporates emotions, considering both current emotional states and lingering feelings (Finucane, 2000). For instance, studies have shown that individuals who are depressed or sad are more likely to predict adverse events. At the same time, those experiencing higher levels of anger tend to anticipate exciting outcomes (DeSteno et al., 2000). Additionally, more anxious individuals are more prone to predicting personal or environmental disasters, such as a stroke or flood, compared to those who are in a state of anger and rage (Lerner & Keltner, 2000). Building on these findings, Paul Slovic (2010), a prominent risk analyst, introduced the concept of 'risk as emotion', which explores how emotions and cognition interact in risk perception. He emphasised that if risks are communicated solely through information without considering emotional aspects, this approach may fail to capture attention and motivate action effectively.

As a result of these insights, a new field has emerged dedicated to understanding the role of emotions in risk perception and behaviour, known as *affect heuristics* (Gigerenzer, 2014; Trujillo, 2018).

Expertise is not just defined by rational or irrational views; it also involves trust, intuition, and emotion. Trust is crucial when risk uncertainty is high (Luhmann, 1993), a topic still debated today. Combining empirical knowledge with intuition and emotion helps navigate uncertainty. Risk estimation isn't purely logical, but rather a mix of rational and irrational strategies, which can lead to probabilistic illusions and dangerous outcomes. Misjudgements influence health behaviours and anxiety. Here are examples of harmful effects from probabilistic illusions in health behaviour and anxiety.

Overestimating rare diseases occurs when people, influenced by vivid anecdotes or media, believe they're at higher risk of a disease after experiencing common symptoms, despite low probability. They may misinterpret false positives in tests, assuming that a positive result indicates disease, like a low-specificity cancer test leading to false alarms. The *availability heuristic* causes overestimation of risk after media coverage. The *gambler's fallacy* leads some to believe they're 'due' for illness after good health, causing obsessive symptom monitoring and misjudging normal sensations (Gigerenzer, 2014).

These examples illustrate how misinterpretations of probabilities and cognitive biases can lead to unhealthy behaviours, overdiagnosis, and health anxiety. Promoting education in health, numeracy, and risk communication is essential for effective prevention. Recently, the internet has made a wealth of health-related information, both accurate and misleading, easily accessible. This has significantly eroded healthcare trust (George, 2024). There has also been a growing interest in risk communication, mainly due to global trends. A significant portion of this communication focuses on health issues and the associated health risks (Fischer, 2024). A recent initiative called the Social Amplification of Risk Framework (SARF) underscores the importance of incorporating sociocultural factors and critical perspectives (Pidgeon et al., 2003). The authors aimed to unify fragmented risk perception and health anxiety models within an integrated framework. This framework spans various disciplines, including media studies, psychometrics, cultural approaches, and organisational studies. It seeks to illustrate the dynamic processes underlying risk perception. A key concept within this framework is *risk amplification,* where a relatively low-risk event garners significant social interest and attention, ultimately influencing health outcomes. Conversely, *risk attenuation* occurs when risks that experts perceive as high are perceived by the public as low.

Assessing the precise level of risk in a specific social situation and communicating that risk to individuals can be challenging and complex tasks (Fischer, 2024). However, there is an increasing demand for predictability regarding these risks at a societal level. Online discussions regarding health and lifestyle risks are also prevalent, as these subjects rank among the most searched online (Bachl et al., 2024). This interest is partly driven by a longstanding desire to explain illness through personal will and actions, as well as the urge to control it through diet, exercise, or other means. However, according to Crawford's (1980) concept of healthism, the aim is not merely to explain illness; rather, Western neoliberal societies increasingly expect moral citizens to take responsibility for their health. In today's consumer society, the array of health-related tools and products in the health industry inundates us with advertisements for various products, some based on scientific evidence and others on pseudoscience, making it difficult to discern which ones are reliable. These advertisements appeal to our desire to feel empowered to take control of our health, often promoting quick-fix solutions or 'miracle cures'.

In media and scientific publications, a continuous stream of probability estimates and statistics regarding health risks is available. How people interpret this information dramatically influences their health behaviours and related anxiety. A prominent example is the widely publicised case of actress Angelina Jolie. After losing her mother, grandmother, and aunt to gynaecological cancer, she underwent genetic testing. This testing showed that she had a mutation in the BRCA1 gene, which indicated an 87% chance of developing breast cancer (Desai & Jena, 2016). To take preventative measures, Angelina Jolie decided to undergo a double mastectomy, which involved the removal of both breasts. Following the operation, she published an article in *The New York Times* to raise awareness among women who might be at risk (Jolie, 2013). She highlighted the importance of prevention and the potential benefits of genetic testing. Two years later, Jolie underwent another surgery to have both her ovaries and fallopian tubes removed after genetic testing revealed a 50% risk of ovarian cancer. News of this operation also garnered significant media attention (Jolie Pitt, 2015). Her initial announcement in 2013 sparked considerable global controversy, making the article one of the most widely read health stories in popular media. In the 15 working days after her announcement, the rate of BRCA genetic testing among women aged 18 to 64 in the United States increased by 64% (Desai & Jena, 2016). Interestingly, the rate of mastectomies performed did not change, indicating that it was not necessarily those who qualified for genetic screening who pursued it, but rather those inspired and engaged by Angelina Jolie's message and who could afford the genetic tests.

This case illustrates that public engagement by celebrities and the sharing of their personal experiences can significantly influence health anxiety and preventive behaviours. However, it also emphasises that such messages may not always resonate with the target audience – in this case, women at risk of breast and ovarian cancer. This discrepancy can be attributed to various social and cultural factors and inequities, including health literacy, access to media and the internet, and the costs associated with screening tests, which could reach $3,000 at that time. Additionally, previous health behaviours, beliefs, attitudes, and questions of autonomy and social justice are significant in this issue. Consequently, it is essential to integrate critical health psychological insights and skills into individual and public health initiatives and personalised intervention planning and care principles (Chamberlain & Lyons, 2022). Moreover, health-related figures can be presented in various ways, eliciting different emotional and behavioural responses. This can benefit some individuals while disadvantaging others, thereby reinforcing power relations and the status quo. Misunderstandings and anxieties can arise if these figures are presented unilaterally and lack sufficient context. For example, in the United States, annual prostate screening was introduced in the 1990s, leading to an increase in the diagnosis of mild, non-progressive cases that had previously gone unnoticed. Several celebrities have shared their personal stories about 'surviving' prostate cancer (Watson, 2023). While survival is a reality for these individuals, it is essential to note that this experience is not directly comparable to cases where different diagnostic tests are performed at later stages of the disease (Takeda, 2017). A similar misleading distinction can be observed in colorectal cancer statistics: although mortality rates are identical, differences in diagnosis timing result in a five-year survival rate of 60% in the United States compared to only 35% in the United Kingdom (Gigerenzer, 2014). This discrepancy highlights that the timing and severity of the diagnosis can significantly impact survival rates.

Estimation errors in risk assessment can also be significantly influenced by various risk denial and neutralisation strategies, which can be viewed as attempts to alleviate anxiety (Breznitz, 1983; Peretti-Watel, 2003). Among these, *denial of personal involvement* is a common response (Covino et al., 2011). Clinical experience, including our own, suggests, for example, that patients in cardiology wards have lowered their own risk of fatal heart attack than their fellow patients by using the 'it cannot happen to me' defence. The following form of denial is the *denial of urgency*. An example of this is when people with severe symptoms do not seek medical attention in time because they deny that they are in serious trouble and need urgent intervention. Similarly, *denial of vulnerability* is common, for example, when it is assumed that doing certain things for one's health, such as taking vitamins or using alternative medicines, will act as a kind of amulet to protect one from even serious illness so that one does not need to be screened or see a doctor. Other examples of unconscious denial occur when one relinquishes individual responsibility and attributes the disease entirely to fate or a stroke of bad luck, or when they close off their consciousness, dismissing all expert information and relying solely on theories devised either by themselves or by sources they trust to be credible and reliable. These psychological strategies to reduce risk perception and anxiety may also partly explain the beliefs and behaviours during the COVID-19 pandemic, such as denial of the virus or vaccine (Fuławka et al., 2024).

Raising awareness of risks among both professionals and the public is essential, particularly if it has a positive impact on health and well-being, rather than being merely for its own sake. To reduce risk behaviours and unnecessary health anxieties, we must communicate scientific information effectively, critically assess media and online sources, and comprehend the complex processes influencing our fears and attitudes towards risk. It is essential to train health communicators who can help the public interpret media messages that may be uninformed, unintentionally distorted, or deliberately misleading. Careful consideration should be given to messages from commercial operators promoting products and services that seek to exploit individuals (and their health concerns) for profit. However, we must also recognise that absolute certainty does not exist. Instead, there is often an illusion of certainty driven by an emotional need for it, and we need to learn how to accept and manage these emotions.

Conclusion

In this chapter, we have traced the evolution of understanding anxiety in psychological and philosophical thought, with a particular emphasis on existential and civilisational anxiety. The concept of late modernity as an 'age of anxiety' has also been introduced, along with the factors shaping perceptions of health threats in our globalised and digitalised world. The diversity of definitions and the fluidity of concepts also show that a thorough and critical approach deserves priority, especially in a time when social media and self-help psychology books promote the idea of living without anxiety, inadvertently increasing health anxiety as a counter-effect. Critically evaluating the dominant individualistic view of anxiety as a mental health issue could foster a comprehensive understanding that requires a multidimensional perspective. For effective prevention and management of different forms of anxiety, including health anxiety, it is essential to recognise that anxiety is a natural part of daily life, capable of leading to both adaptive and adverse outcomes. A relatively new yet essential topic that extends beyond its research significance is the impact of consumer society and media, particularly social media, on health anxiety, intolerance of uncertainty, and MHW. Further detailed investigation is necessary to understand how perceptions and assessments of health-related risks, along with rational, emotional, and sociocultural factors, contribute to anxiety. The importance of responsible, credible, and transparent scientific communication about health risks conveyed by the media cannot be overstated, as it promotes equitable access to healthcare and enhances autonomy in health decision-making.

2

HEALTH CONCERNS IN RISK SOCIETIES

In the previous chapter, we discussed anxiety and the concept of living in an 'age of anxiety', as proposed by psychological and social science theories. In recent decades, there has been a growing emphasis on the role of emotions, particularly in relation to societal fears and uncertainties. This shift has not only underscored the importance of predominantly negative emotions but has also introduced a new methodology, *affect heuristics*, for the scientific examination of health-related risks and concerns (Trujillo, 2018). This perspective is also linked to the broader social theory idea that modern societies are becoming increasingly emotionally oriented, as the means to express, communicate, share, and manipulate emotional responses have become more accessible through mass communication and social media (Jacobsen, 2021). The shift is also due to the prevalent belief that we are facing complex and turbulent times. This perspective focuses on the current shift in collective awareness and its impact on the formation of health risk perceptions, which also play a significant role in shaping emotional responses. The change has furthermore resulted in a shift in focus from a narrow psychological perspective to a more historical, social, and cultural context. Consequently, new fields such as the sociology of emotions and the transdisciplinary approach in health risk studies have emerged as distinct research areas in recent decades (Bericat, 2016; Giritli-Nygren & Olofson, 2014).

The influential work on the process of civilisation by Norbert Elias (2000) has inspired researchers to emphasise that the interdisciplinary study of emotions can provide a way of analysing contemporary society, including individualisation, globalisation, digitalisation, and consumerism, among other social processes, in more detail (van Krieken, 2014). Furthermore, it allows for an exploration of the question raised by social scientists regarding the possible correlation between the increasing mechanisation of society through commodification, commercialisation,

DOI: 10.4324/9781003517788-2

digitalisation, manipulation, and distortion, and the industrialisation of collective emotions (Meštrović, 1997). This prompts the question of whether it is possible to argue that emotions and risk perception in our contemporary society are becoming 'synthetic', detached from experience, which may result in a reduction in solidarity and compassion, or whether, as other scholars have suggested, there is an increase in emotional orientation. The latter group of scholars has argued that the dominant emotional patterns in contemporary society are defensive and negative emotions, including anxiety, stress, depression, apathy, fear, hatred, and nostalgia (Jacobsen, 2021). The argument has been made that these emotions have become so pervasive in today's digitalised societies that people cannot often distinguish between real, imagined, or artificially created sources of fear. The concept of 'liquid fear', which refers to the pervasive and ever-changing nature of fear, was introduced by sociologist Zygmunt Bauman (2006). In his subsequent concept of 'liquid modernity', he argued that society does not provide individuals with adequate security, resulting in uncertainty about their self-identity (Bauman, 2017). This may be attributed to the extreme complexity of our contemporary world and the pervasive awareness of crises through media and internet-based sources. Moreover, concerns regarding the uncertainties of self-identity can give rise to fears of bodily vulnerability, which may, in turn, precipitate the onset of health anxiety. It can also be posited that defensive emotions and related nostalgia function as a form of psychological defence against fear, providing a means of controlling and anchoring free-floating anxiety.

The significance of health as a value for both the individual and the society renders it an optimal medium for both the projection and the anchoring of fears. This raises the question of the veracity, authenticity, and constructed nature of individual and societal concerns about various threats, particularly those related to health. The issues discussed in this chapter, encompassing the social and scientific discourse on eco-anxiety and the perceived health risks associated with the COVID-19 pandemic, underscore the inherent complexity of the problem. However, at the individual level, most concerns pertain to the body's safety. In recent years, numerous critical theorists have extensively referred to the concept of 'biopolitics', as developed by Michel Foucault (2008). These theorists have argued that the body has emerged as a significant concern in late modernity (Russo, 2020). Since the 20th century, the body has been described as being vulnerable in professional and everyday discourse, necessitating constant protection and monitoring (Campbell & Sitze, 2013). The concept of safety has assumed heightened significance within postmodern societies. In addition to the persistent threat of war, potential epidemic outbreaks, and the looming spectre of climate change, there has been a notable decline in trust in institutions, governments, and the political process. This has heightened the emphasis on personal and bodily safety as well as on health protection (Perry, 2021).

In the context of the information society, personal anxieties are increasingly manifest in the public sphere. Moreover, heightened self-awareness and self-centredness may emanate from a culture of narcissism, as evidenced by the

American historian and social critic Christopher Lasch (1979) in his seminal work *The Culture of Narcissism*. Some of Lasch's conclusions remain pertinent in the present era, and there is substantial evidence that individuals in the contemporary period frequently perceive the world as a reflection of their fears and desires. It is perhaps unsurprising that narcissism has become a topic of interest in recent years within the field of psychology (Kwon, 2023; Twenge & Campbell, 2009). The increasing self-centredness inevitably influences our perception of environmental risks and our conceptualisation of potential threats to our physical and mental well-being. However, interpreting any situation is always preceded by the perception of the associated risks. As also discussed in the previous chapter, attitudes towards and judgements about risk are situated within a network of cultural relations, expectations, and values specific to various groups (Lupton, 2013). Furthermore, the perception of expertise, scientific reliability, and credibility of risk messages relies on the context in which they are created and disseminated (Nagler et al., 2023; Pallavi et al., 2022).

Symbolic representations of societal anxieties

Societal factors significantly influence risk perception, impacting both perceived and actual health and safety risks. Critical social theory posits that people frequently attribute symbolic meanings to social and natural phenomena to establish order and comprehension (Wilkinson, 2009). This concept was introduced by Mary Douglas (1966), who is widely considered a key figure in the cultural theory of risk and is recognised as the pioneer of this approach. Douglas proposed that social groups tend to develop coherent theories regarding misfortune. By examining the beliefs and behaviours about the danger of tribes in natural settings, she proposed that 'danger' taboos of pollution and contamination are established to maintain social order. This line of thought, particularly the use of symbolic reasoning to justify the protection of society from 'outsiders' and the maintenance of 'order' due to anxieties, has been employed to explain, for example, perceptions of water contamination at different historical points. In medieval Europe, the consumption of poor-quality drinking water constituted a constant and tangible threat to public health. However, when accusations emerged in the 14th century of Jews poisoning wells, the issue took on a political dimension.

The issue of 'harmful' drinking water has also emerged as a reflection of contemporary fears. In the 1970s, the idea that tap water is not truly beneficial to health began to gain traction in Western media and public discourse (Doria, 2006). Such claims were sometimes made without any evidence suggesting poor water quality in the areas from which the water was sourced. Nonetheless, there was a marked shift in consumer behaviour, with an increase in bottled water consumption, leading to the rise of a significant industry catering to this demand (Race, 2012). However, there is growing concern that the production and consumption of bottled water contribute to environmental pollution. Recent discussions have even suggested that mineral water could be more harmful to health than tap water (De Giglio, 2015). Over the years, various parties have contributed to this evolving discourse, including industry representatives, public health professionals, media members, and restaurant chains. In these discussions, fear has frequently been employed as a persuasive tool, with arguments based on health concerns and moral behaviour linked to environmental protection. As an additional illustration of unconscious collective fears, when HIV infection was initially linked to homosexual contact in the 1980s, the perceived danger was attributed to a socially marginalised group, symbolically excluding its members and the infection associated with them from the community (Chambers et al., 2015).

Mary Douglas (1992) posited that the concept of risk in contemporary societies has supplanted culpability, which was prevalent in earlier social orders. There has been a notable shift in attitudes towards health risks in recent decades. This shift has been driven by an increased awareness of health issues, which has led to changes in health-related behaviours, beliefs, and attitudes. Nevertheless, the concept of 'healthism' cautioned against an undue emphasis on individual conduct as the predominant health hazard as early as the 1980s. It was proposed that such an approach may result in attributing blame for their health status to individuals, viewing them as both the aggressor and the victim (Crawford, 1980). Chapter 6 will examine the connection between attributing blame and one's health, as well as perceived societal threats. The role of moralising in public discourse on health remains significant because the uncertainty that pervades contemporary societies often fosters a climate in which health warnings, danger signals, and risk management rituals shape individuals' actions (Kraaijeveld & Jamrozik, 2022). Additionally, there is an unconscious intention to supplant previous moral norms. This emphasis on responsibility and culpability can be counterproductive, rather than providing an empathetic understanding of the factors contributing to risky behaviours and the necessity of presenting options for change and support.

The question of who is authorised to determine risk is very important. In contemporary societies, the dominant message is that individuals, even those with expert knowledge, may lack the capacity to assess risk due to the inherent complexity of the information involved. Consequently, different institutions and authority figures assume responsibility for risk management, and there is a possibility that they may manipulate and distort information for their benefit (Lupton, 1993). For example, the media frequently prioritise sensationalism and simplicity when disseminating information and advertising to reach a wider audience. Relying solely on the media as a source of information can lead to confusion and anxiety, as the messages conveyed are often contradictory, inaccurate, and rooted in existing societal fears.

The pursuit of evidence and certainty

In traditional societies, religion has historically been the main institution through which anxiety was given meaning. In the contemporary era, there is a tendency to seek scientific expertise to confirm or refute fear-inducing health messages. However, scientists do not necessarily occupy a prominent position in the public sphere and frequently lack the communication skills to convey their message effectively (Shah et al., 2022). Health warnings and scare stories often start with 'Researchers have proven that'. While new concerns are discussed, verifying their truth is challenging, partly because many actors, including Big Industry, experts, media, and social platforms, spread these fears. This makes the idea of an ideal health state uncertain, leading to anxiety and risky behaviours. Amid vast information, people seek clear explanations; doubt and scepticism are viewed negatively, though they are vital to science. Today, the public often sees scepticism as a lack of confidence and dismisses claims without evidence (Contessa, 2023; Hornsey, 2020). A significant proportion of the population feels discomfort when uncertain about their health and safety and tends to seek a definitive answer. This desire for certainty, combined with the influence of the media, has led some experts to assume the role of 'truth-tellers', obligated to provide absolute truths. The media often favour straightforward, unequivocal terminology and encounter difficulties conveying intricate or ambiguous data in a manner perceived as favourable. Consequently, it is challenging for the typical media consumer to distinguish between high-quality, well-evaluated health information and less reliable sources. It is also essential to consider the objective of the communication: is it to provide information or to persuade? Furthermore, it is crucial to ponder who is responsible for verifying specific information. In this instance, the communication source will intentionally or unintentionally employ psychological techniques to exert influence. Such techniques may include reliance on emotions, fears, anxieties, and guilt in health behaviour, with questionable results (Moussaoui et al., 2021).

It is commonly assumed by health professionals that clear and understandable risk communication consistently has a significant impact; however, this assumption overlooks ethical considerations and power dynamics. The communication of risk is frequently structured hierarchically. Those in positions of authority, such as media representatives and health policymakers, can control the information disseminated to those lower in the hierarchy (Lupton, 2023). Nevertheless, this may give rise to questions and resistance from the public. One common critique is whether the minority should prioritise the majority's interests in health-related behaviours. Additionally, it is essential to note that professionals often communicate risks to the public using a risk-focused approach rather than a safety-focused, benefit-risk framework (Hampel, 2006). However, research shows that messages framed around benefits and risks are more effective when there is a strong level of trust between the communicator and the audience (Tanemura et al., 2022). Furthermore, statistical data are often presented in terms of risk, which can cause anxiety if not communicated effectively. This anxiety, when suppressed, can impede behavioural change because the person uses the energy required for it to manage anxiety. This may result in risk-taking behaviours and a deterioration in health (Chapman et al., 2013).

Health promotion messages aim to prevent lifestyle-related diseases by influencing people's habits. Opponents have argued that poorly planned and executed programmes in the food, cosmetics, and other 'body industries' can lead to feelings of anxiety and guilt about not engaging in healthy behaviours (Ruiter et al., 2014). These concerns are often overlooked in public discussions in which health is presented as an unquestionable universal good that everyone deserves. The influence of power relations and disciplinary intentions is considered less significant when the primary objective is to promote and develop health. Problems may arise when the hidden agenda of the communication is not to provide support, as it seems, but instead to impose discipline or to undermine health messages by the industry. Conversely, problems can arise when communication lacks expressions of support or suggestions on how to provide help. As a result, the recipients may feel abandoned and possibly even guilty about their inability to change their unhealthy habits.

Risk awareness and the methods of bringing about change in risk behaviour are significantly influenced by an understanding of the risk perceptions and attitudes of a specific social group or individual (Lupton, 1994). These are characterised by a high degree of complexity, with numerous factors, including health literacy, trust, efficacy, and emotional factors, influencing the subtleties (Shi et al., 2023). Nevertheless, discernible patterns can be identified. These can be interpreted, for example, following the classical Grid-Group Cultural Theory typology proposed by Mary Douglas (1982), which categorises worldview types as 'fatalistic', 'hierarchical', 'individualistic', and 'equality seeking'. Multiple studies have investigated these common response patterns concerning health risks and other perceptions of risk (Cambardella et al., 2020; O'Riordan et al., 1997; Zeng et al., 2022). The findings indicate that 'fatalists' perceive risk as an intrinsic aspect of contemporary life, characterised by complexity and uncertainty. Such individuals tend to adopt a negative outlook regarding the potential for positive change in public health. They believe that statistical data can be manipulated and that individuals are best served by exercising their judgement. Those with a hierarchical worldview emphasise the necessity for risk communication to be grounded in empirical evidence rather than imposed from above. Individualists assert that it is the individual's responsibility to acquire relevant information, yet they also contend that this should be achieved through social networks. Those with egalitarian views perceive risk as an intrinsic aspect of social anxiety and posit that societal transformation and democratisation are prerequisites for change. The findings confirm that, if there is a significant difference in knowledge between the source and the recipient of health risk information, the information will only be effective if the recipient sees the source as credible and accepts the information. Otherwise, the dissemination of health advice will be perceived as an authoritarian command. The relationship between the individual and the authority figure, whether the government, experts, or the media, is a significant factor in the risk perception. This relationship is not static but can change (Kington et al., 2021). This is particularly pertinent in the context of what has been termed 'risk societies' in the present era.

Perceived threats inside and outside

Sociologist Ulrich Beck's monograph *Risk Society: Towards a New Modernity* (1992) marked a significant milestone in the study of risk perception. It coincided with the Chernobyl disaster, providing concrete evidence to support Beck's concept of the 'risk society'. In this seminal work, Beck posited that the exclusive emphasis on technological advancement in classical modernisation was becoming untenable. He emphasised the need for better readiness for the upcoming significant changes in society and lifestyle, expected with the rise of the information society and the knowledge-based economy. Its innovative approach enhanced the understanding of modern social dynamics by focusing on the concept of risk rather than traditional categories such as class, gender, economy, and power (Mythen, 2021). This theory emphasised anticipated threats over current crises, making it particularly useful for exploring health risk perception and the social factors that influence health and ecological anxiety.

Beck developed the concept of *reflexive modernisation* in collaboration with Anthony Giddens and Scott Lash, with a particular focus on ecological processes (Beck et al., 1994). The concept posits that we are in a transitional phase, moving from a primarily natural to a primarily social-risk environment. Such circumstances have the potential to precipitate extreme stress and anxiety, which in turn may elevate health risks. The dissolution of communities is a contributing factor to a decline in mental health, which in turn gives rise to increased anxiety and addiction. This situation has the potential to impede the continued development and advancement of modernisation.

Furthermore, Beck (1992) emphasised the importance of several key dichotomies. One such contrast between certainty and uncertainty is increasingly difficult to define, given the inherent challenge of determining the concept of certainty itself. The tension between these dichotomies represents a significant source of anxiety. The second dichotomy is between the concepts of 'inside' and 'outside'. As evidenced by the recent COVID-19 pandemic and the increasingly apparent climate crisis, threats to health and security are no longer constrained by geographical boundaries, thereby blurring the dichotomy between 'inside' and 'outside'. In Beck's view, the interconnectedness of the modern world, brought about by globalisation, means that threats can emerge from anywhere. Nevertheless, the absence of an apparent threat makes it difficult to ascertain the level of risk.

It is a well-established tenet of social psychology that individuals frequently seek to regulate their emotions and mitigate their sense of threat by constructing simplifications and stereotypes. One such simplification is reinforcing the dichotomy between friend and foe, whereby anxieties about the 'stranger', the hostile, dangerous 'Other', are aroused (Staszak, 2009). In the contemporary era, the human being responsible for destroying the Earth's resources has also become a 'dangerous Other' in collective representations. This generates considerable anxiety, as evidenced by the discourse that this 'Other' is, in fact, us and that we do not adequately value nature (Albrecht, 2019). This creates a challenging conflict as individuals are both victims of and responsible for behaviours that damage their health or the environment. The greater an individual's acceptance of the concept of a risk society and their consideration of the world in terms of risk, the higher the probability that they will experience internal conflicts regarding the acceptability of specific risks (Wilkinson, 2009). For example, one of the primary sociopolitical disputes during the COVID-19 pandemic can be distilled into a fundamental dichotomy: the potential adverse effects of quarantine, such as economic, mental, relational, and other risks to individuals, versus the peril of unchecked infection and its concomitant consequences.

There is a debate in both professional and lay discourse regarding the merits of maintaining a state of constant risk awareness and whether such a state may cause excessive anxiety (Nakayachi, 2013). However, this can be beneficial insofar as risk awareness facilitates the development of coping mechanisms, thereby reducing anxiety. The most significant risk associated with crisis communication is the potential for panic and a lack of transparency and trust, which can significantly increase uncertainty. Moreover, the dissemination of contradictory information from multiple sources, the delayed release of pertinent data, the display of paternalistic attitudes, and the lack of a prompt response to rumours may exacerbate this phenomenon (Reynolds & Seeger, 2005). Such factors may also have influenced the circumstances that unfolded in northern Italy at the onset of the coronavirus outbreak in 2020. The high mortality rate at the outset of the initial phase of the epidemic was attributed by numerous commentators to shortcomings in Italian mass communication. It was posited that this should serve as a cautionary tale for other countries (Ruiu, 2020). Analysts have suggested that numerous political issues exist between the central and regional governments, the government and scientists, and the government and the public. These also led to many individuals becoming distrustful of the measures implemented and, as a result, failing to comply, which inadvertently contributed to the unintentional spread of the virus. Concurrently, individuals hailing from the afflicted regions were subjected to domestic and international social stigma. In a CNN broadcast, Italy was held responsible for the global crisis. A map titled 'Coronavirus Cases Linked to Italy' was published, and it employed red arrows to indicate that the virus had disseminated 'everywhere' from Italy (ANSA, 2020). The messages from multiple sources, which the media even played up to contradict themselves, led many people to ignore the warning messages and thus became the starting point for infections.

A common feature of public messages on both the coronavirus pandemic and the climate crisis, both global crises, is the attribution of blame to external forces (Krämer & Winkler, 2024). There has been a tendency in both the media and public discourse to portray the pandemic and global warming as 'Nature's backlash', whereby Nature is perceived as punishing humans for their perceived neglect and destruction of the natural environment. According to the cultural anthropological theory put forth by Douglas and Wildawsky (1982), the concept of God in modern societies has been supplanted by that of Nature. Following this line of reasoning, the reclamation of Nature in contemporary vernacular discourse may also symbolically imply that global consumer societies have appropriated the divine rather than the natural and that humanity, perceived as inherently sinful, deserves punishment. This symbolic representation may serve to reduce feelings of insecurity and anxiety by providing a focus for fears that may otherwise remain unresolved. Conversely, it can be a deliberate or inadvertent instrument of retributive justice, enabling individuals to ascribe culpability to those whom they perceive to have precipitated the peril. A potentially positive outcome of this discourse is that it may also strengthen solidarity among marginalised, vulnerable, or anti-consumption groups in consumer societies, as a common threat unites disparate individuals around a shared goal. Nevertheless, whether global goals can be discussed in general terms is a matter of debate. One of the most common criticisms of Beck's risk society theory is that it presents a monolithic concept of risk, failing to acknowledge the existence of other global issues (Jarvis, 2007). Furthermore, as critics have asserted, the notion of a 'world risk society' implies that hazards and risks are distributed uniformly (Rasborg, 2012). Significant disparities exist in this domain across the globe, as do considerable inequalities in the extent to which the level of concern about a given hazard is perceived to be realistic (Mythen, 2021).

It is a historicist question whether individuals in contemporary global societies, often characterised by heightened levels of anxiety and insecurity, experience greater feelings of these emotions than those in the past. Nonetheless, the rise of media and internet platforms has made it increasingly common for individuals to openly express their anxiety in the modern era (De Lemos, 2016). As discussed in the previous chapter, some commentators have suggested that this may serve to reinforce fear and contribute to the emergence of a culture of anxiety in the 'age of anxiety' (Furedi, 2007). In such arguments, the media are held responsible for this phenomenon, claiming that there was less news, fewer adverse events, and less information about dangers in previous eras. This assertion is refuted by evidence indicating that ambivalence and concerns about the impact of the media emerged as early as the 19th century, with the advent of the press and the growth of journalism (Drotner, 1999). The key issue here is the purpose of disseminating content that induces fear. The question thus arises as to whether the dissemination of fear-inducing content is intended to inform, serve business interests, gain popularity, or process anxiety and trigger self-reflection. Furthermore, how individual and collective forms of anxiety interact and influence mental well-being and health-related behaviours necessitates further investigation. In this context, particularly, given the challenges posed by the climate crisis, we are all engaged in a global 'field study' of our times.

Eco-anxiety and health issues in context

Anxiety about climate change is a pervasive collective phenomenon in our time and a major contributor to health concerns. A recent international Google statistics report indicated that, during the initial 10 months of 2023, there were 27 times as many searches for 'climate anxiety' and 'eco-anxiety' in English than in 2017 (Moench, 2023). In Portuguese, the increase was even more substantial, reaching 73 times the previous level. This trend is particularly noteworthy among the younger demographic. A comprehensive global survey of 10,000 respondents revealed that 59% of young people worldwide reported experiencing intense or extreme anxiety about the future, pollution, and climate change (Hickman et al., 2021). Moreover, 84% of respondents reported suffering at least moderate anxiety, accompanied by feelings of fear, helplessness, guilt, and anger. It has been established that such issues can give rise to a range of health concerns, including eating disorders and severe motivational disorders, the influence of which can be shaped by public communication. The *WHO* has long acknowledged the impact of climate change on physical and mental health (Costello et al., 2009). Several concepts have emerged to describe the various emotions, feelings, and mental states related to climate change. These are collectively known as 'climate emotions', 'ecological emotions', or 'ecological distress' (Cianconi et al., 2023). Furthermore, the term 'psychoterratic syndromes' has been put forth to describe circumstances in which an individual's mental well-being is shaped by the interconnection between the Earth and the environment and by the individual's mental processes and overall health (Albrecht, 2011).

In recent years, the concept of eco-anxiety has become a significant topic of discussion both within the scientific community and in everyday conversations. However, there is still no agreement on the exact definition of the term (Niedzwiedz & Katikireddi, 2023). Some have suggested that eco-anxiety is a stress reaction to ecosystem disruption caused by climate change, while others argue it is an anxiety disorder connected to worries about environmental decline and the risk of ecological catastrophe (Mento et al., 2023). However, scholars have agreed that as people become more aware of the potential consequences of climate change, they are likely to see this information, consciously or unconsciously, as threatening and to feel emotions such as anxiety, sadness, anger, shame, or grief (Albrecht, 2019). The most prevalent of these are anxiety and worry. Although these responses may be innate and potentially adaptive, there is also a strong tendency in Western societies to medicalise and pathologise them (Christodoulou et al., 2024b). Furthermore, it can result in the attribution of victimhood to those affected, which can, in turn, lead to additional health anxiety, feelings of loneliness, self-blame, and mental health issues. For example, a review study found a correlation between elevated levels of eco-anxiety and the presence of depression, anxiety, post-traumatic stress disorder (PTSD), distress, sleep disturbances, diminished self-evaluation of mental health, and reluctance to have children (Boluda-Verdú et al., 2022). However, evaluating the methodology and theoretical approach used to support such correlations is crucial. For example, a new multidimensional scale has been developed to supersede the previous Climate Anxiety Scale (Clayton & Karazsia, 2020). The four factors of the new measure (affective symptoms, rumination, behavioural symptoms, and anxiety regarding personal impact on the planet) do not address social and cultural dimensions (Hogg et al., 2021). The instrument is oriented mainly towards the assessment of symptoms previously determined by the researchers, like of depression, stress, and anxiety.

Having reliable tools with diverse approaches, including in-depth qualitative measures, for identifying and understanding mental health problems is of paramount importance. It is also imperative to consider how the clinical focus of research is reflected in public discourse and thinking. A news report from *Euronews* and other news outlets underscored the need to examine meticulously the influence of expert and non-expert discourses on eco-anxiety in the media and online. The report outlined the tragic suicide of a 30-year-old Belgian man who had engaged in conversation with the chatbot ELIZA (Atillah, 2023). It was alleged that ELIZA had encouraged him to take his own life to save the planet. While mental health issues or other factors may have influenced the suicide, how such reports are presented in the media could contribute to an increase in anxiety. For example, in 2018, the media framed the suicide of human rights lawyer and climate activist David Buckel as a 'climate suicide' (Ray, 2020).

It is indisputable that the global climate crisis represents a significant and growing threat, highlighting the necessity for communication on the subject to be both informative and constructive. In September 2020, *The Lancet*, the pre-eminent medical journal, published a call to action, emphasising that the stress associated with the global climate crisis affects children and young people (Wu et al., 2020). The authors highlighted the likelihood of increased incidence of mental health issues over a lifetime because of repeated exposure to climate-related stressors. The authors proposed that chronic stress during adolescence can lead to long-lasting alterations in brain structure in later life. The cohort, known as Generation Z, has experienced the climate crisis throughout its entire lifespan. The term 'climate generation' has been coined to describe this cohort's potential for effecting change and their longer lifespan (Ray, 2020). However, such labelling, primarily due to the influence of social media, can contribute to the construction of young people's identities, changes in their emotional states, and even the formation of symptoms. Nevertheless, despite the connectivity of the internet, this generation is more susceptible to feelings of loneliness, anxiety, and depression (Léger-Goodes et al., 2022). In a recent study by Petrescu-Mag et al. (2023), Millennials and Generation Z perceived themselves as 'observers' rather than 'players' concerning climate change and perceived health threats. The study demonstrated that they did not anticipate engaging in efforts to address these issues. In response to this situation, *UNICEF* (2022) initiated a 'Climate Heroes' programme to support action, its primary responsibility being to investigate perceptions and beliefs and to foster awareness of the issue.

In a review study analysing communications from 2012 to 2022, researchers identified a correlation between elevated levels of climate change perception and awareness and an increased prevalence of depression, anxiety, adjustment disorders, stress, and addictive behaviours (Gianfredi et al., 2024). In an editorial published in April 2024 in *Nature*, the findings of a study of 16 to 25-year-olds in 10 countries were presented (Editorial, 2024). The study revealed that 45% of respondents indicated that climate change affects their daily lives, work, and sleep. Furthermore, it was noted that most of the previous research has been conducted in more developed countries and has primarily focused on investigating clinical-level issues, such as severe anxiety, depression, and suicide risk. Conversely, a considerable proportion of the global population resides in countries where the ratio of psychiatrists to the population is less than 1 per 200,000 inhabitants. This underscores the issue that a substantial number of mental health concerns, at least as these are defined by Western knowledge systems and mental health nomenclature, remain undetected. The authors emphasised the necessity of prevention, and the available evidence (mainly from Western studies) indicates that people feel helpless and abandoned. Therefore, it is essential to adopt coping strategies, support those affected, and gain a detailed understanding of the differences in cultural contexts.

It is promising, however, that a cross-national survey conducted years ago, which included participants from the United States, Canada, and Malta, found that residents of these countries demonstrated an increased awareness of the vulnerability of people in developing nations (Akerlof et al., 2010). Additionally, respondents believed that climate change could lead to the emergence of severe chronic diseases, allergies, infectious diseases, and accidents. It is important to note that the responses regarding health risks were elicited through prompted questions, whereas these concerns were less prominent in the responses to open-ended questions. This raises the question of whether these anxieties were not fully conscious or not as strong as they appeared to be in the direct questions. This finding also emphasises the significance of qualitative research in obtaining insight and understanding.

In an Australian study, perceived health risks associated with climate change were found to be related to, but distinct from, an individual's risk to self and society (Arnot et al., 2024). A survey conducted in Germany yielded comparable results. Most respondents (83%) perceived a potential detrimental impact of climate change on health. However, the level of perceived risk exhibited by the respondents was lower (69%) than that reported by the global population (89%), as indicated by van Baal et al. (2023). The tendency to avoid cognitive dissonance appears to have played a role in this, despite Germany being considered a safer option. The phenomenon of cognitive dissonance may also account for the finding that, in Canada, individuals tended to perceive the harm associated with drinking water or air quality as a more significant concern (Casson et al., 2023). However, this perception was also influenced by sociodemographic variables, with women, those with higher education, and those with a left-wing political orientation demonstrating more significant concern about health risks. The role of socio-economic variables, such as higher education, in health risk perception was also confirmed in a study conducted among Brazilian farmers (de Moura et al., 2023). Furthermore, the study by Petrescu-Mag and colleagues (2022) revealed intriguing cross-cultural contrasts. The respondents from Belgium were found to ascribe responsibility for climate change to individuals, whereas those from Romania attributed it to large companies, governments, and consumers.

Emotions as catalysts for action

Professionals must be careful to avoid pathologising, labelling, or stigmatising different eco-emotions without signs of clinical anxiety. Instead, these should be seen as a form of anxiety that can be described as 'practical anxiety' (Pihkala, 2021). This form of anxiety prompts individuals to seek information and reassess their behaviour when faced with uncertainty. Similarly, Verlie (2022) proposed that eco-anxiety should be regarded as a catalyst for action, drawing upon the etymological meaning of emotion to move outward. Consequently, rather than focusing on treating or curing climate distress, it is possible to consider the action potential that emotions can facilitate. Individuals must be provided with the necessary support to accept the inevitability of addressing climate change (and the associated anxiety) as a fundamental reality. Some commentators advocate for the importance of 'deep adaptation', which encompasses non-violence, respect, openness, and compassion, as a constructive framework for addressing anxieties about the threat of societal collapse due to the climate crisis (Bendell & Read, 2021). Others suggested that while eco-anxiety can significantly impede appropriate environmental behaviour, it may be alleviated by altering risk perception, attitudes, and perceived behaviour control (Arya & Kumar, 2023). Moreover, they emphasised the importance of this in the context of psychoeducation.

Health professionals must undergo training, as international studies have demonstrated that, although they recognise the significant health impacts of climate change, their understanding of the issue is still lacking (Hathaway & Maibach, 2018). In education, it is also imperative to emphasise that climate risk is not an isolated, individual phenomenon but rather an emotional response to a threat that affects humanity. It is, therefore, essential to expand the traditional psychological interpretive framework with a socio-economic dimension. This represents an undertaking in social psychology and critical social theory (Davidson, 2023). The message emphasises that framing responses to climate change as an individualised and medicalised psychological issue trivialises the problem and perpetuates a system that maintains power. This may be why, in many cases, individuals choose to disregard institutional risk assessments, instead relying on their instincts, past experiences, and tolerance (Alaszewski, 2005). This is, at least in part, due to deficiencies in communication, as there is no established protocol for sharing information about global health crises with the public. The deficiencies in communication regarding the global situation concerning the coronavirus have also resulted from the general unavailability of such expert teams and the lack of attention paid to their involvement (Mihelj et al., 2022).

The field of health risk communication has historically focused on disseminating information about specific disease-related behavioural risks such as the likelihood of developing heart disease or cancer. This approach has primarily concentrated on communicating individual health risk behaviours, with messages directed at individuals rather than the public. As a result, there is a lack of trained professionals in social communication. As previously discussed, the tendency of the news media to prioritise storytelling over the dissemination of responsible information is a matter of particular concern. This has been the foundation for numerous misunderstandings and challenges in public health initiatives, as evidenced by the West Nile virus, the earlier severe acute respiratory syndrome (SARS) epidemic, and the measles epidemic (Sauvayre, 2021). Nevertheless, a frequently asked question is whether the media should be held accountable to the same normative standards during crises as other institutions involved in disease management and prevention. This naturally gives rise to several broader ethical and societal questions about democracy. However, there is a strong consensus that a significantly enhanced level of collaboration should exist among news media, social media, digital technologies, experts, and various institutions. This collaboration can be facilitated, for instance, by social psychologists, health psychologists, other professionals, a range of non-governmental organisations (NGOs), and individuals who are more directly involved in common issues and who take personal responsibility for their health and seek autonomy.

Conclusion

To examine how living in contemporary 'risk societies' affects our health behaviours and anxieties, a comprehensive perspective has been proposed. This chapter has explored theories of symbolic representations, critical social theory, and the concept of 'defensive emotions', considering how fear and uncertainty – arising from both real and perceived threats – influence our perception of health risks. A significant example of this is the global reactions to COVID-19 and the widespread ecological anxiety observed today, which connects with health anxiety and mental health challenges among climate-conscious individuals and younger generations. These concerns underscore the crucial role of trust in experts and scientific narratives, as well as their impact on health anxiety. However, it is essential to recognise that emotions like anxiety can serve as both barriers and motivators for action and coping when managed effectively. The research highlighted in the chapter emphasises that acknowledging moderate worry as a normal response to environmental threats is key. Moreover, there should be a focus on the long-term experience and management of defensive emotions, along with the coping strategies adopted in response. The first step involves identifying the specific nature of the emotions at play rather than hastily labelling them as pathological anxiety.

3

FROM HYPOCHONDRIA TO HEALTH EMPOWERMENT

Occasionally, we all feel anxious about physical sensations or symptoms, even without experiencing them, but this is usually temporary and does not affect our daily lives. However, there is a level of anxiety about health and illness that disrupts normal life and habits. In everyday language, this is often called hypochondria, a term first used by the ancient Greeks to describe anxiety about illness and symptoms (Baur, 1989). This concept, which has undergone numerous transformations, has accompanied the history of medicine, and these transformations have also reflected the uncertainty and anxiety of both lay people and professionals regarding the body and symptoms whose origin was unknown (Crampton, 2024). The term 'hypochondria' itself – hypochondriasis in medical terminology – was initially associated by the ancient Greeks with the hypochondrium, the area of the body located below the lower ribs and in the abdomen. Hippocrates and his contemporaries had different ideas about this area, seeing it as the source of symptoms that were difficult to explain. This was partly because it was not until the Renaissance that dissection made it possible to see inside the body. At that time, the uterus, which had been thought to move around the body for centuries and cause various symptoms, was also considered important in interpreting medically unexplained symptoms in women (Shetty et al., 2020). Thus, the concept of hysteria was developed, overlapping with hypochondria, with an intense stigmatisation of the symptoms. This was primarily due to the perceived 'feminine' nature of the symptoms, which were also associated with attributes of fear of the unknown (Cleghorn, 2021; Jordanova, 1993). From the 17th century onwards, Enlightenment physicians sought to remove hypochondria and hysteria from their status as 'mysteries', to medicalise and neutralise them, and to see them as a kind of inherited vulnerability that the affected individual (woman) had to live with. From the end of the 19th century, with the

DOI: 10.4324/9781003517788-3

emergence of psychiatry and psychoanalysis, professionals returned to dealing with psychopathological forms of hypochondriasis rather than everyday health anxiety (Crampton, 2024; Gilman et al., 1993). From the mid-20th century, hypochondriasis as pathology and health anxiety as a more general phenomenon came back to the fore, partly with the emergence of psychosomatic medicine and later health psychology. This is partly because the number of medically unexplained symptoms has not decreased despite rapid advancements in medical science. According to the *WHO*, many patients still present to specialists with unexplained symptoms, ranging from 30% to 40% (Vermeir et al., 2021). However, providing precise figures is challenging due to uncertainties in definitions and diagnoses. Different studies have reported a wide variation in the prevalence of medically unexplained symptoms, ranging from 2.9% to 76% (Jadhakhan et al., 2022). Regardless, these symptoms continue to cause significant anxiety for those affected and often lead to frustration in the doctor-patient relationship. In many cases, even when doctors try to approach these symptoms through a complex, psychosocial perspective, patients feel stigmatised by the questioning of the 'reality' of their symptoms and by psychological explanations. This is due to not only negative stereotypes about mental problems but also the age-old stigma of hypochondria and hysteria.

The term hypochondria, along with hysteria, which has been linked to femininity, has long been seen as a stigma, the sign of moral weakness, or mental illness in everyday language throughout medical history (Crampton, 2024). It was not until 1980 that hysteria was removed from official medical terminology, and not until 2013 that hypochondriasis was also removed. Despite the much lower prevalence of clinical-level health anxiety, the colloquial use of hypochondria persists. Pathological forms known as illness anxiety disorder or somatic symptom disorder significantly interfere with daily life and cause considerable distress. This requires the simultaneous fulfilment of the following criteria: (1) preoccupation with symptoms or illness, (2) fear of illness, (3) assumption of illness, (4) misinterpretation of physical symptoms, and (5) persistent worry despite medical examination and reassurance. According to recent surveys, the prevalence ranges from 0.04% to 4.5% in the general population (Bailey, 2024). However, the prevalence of health anxiety not considered pathological is much higher (up to around 20%), and surveys suggest it is increasing (Kosic et al., 2020; Tyrer et al., 2019). There is no clear consensus on when health anxiety reaches a clinically significant level. Still, there is no doubt that the problem places a heavy burden on both individuals and health systems worldwide (Hannah et al., 2023).

Uncertainties in classification

The definitions of health anxiety, illness anxiety, and hypochondria have always been quite ambiguous. In the first half of the 20th century, 18 different everyday and medical applications of hypochondria were described. These ranged from general anxiety about the body and illness to anxiety; neurasthenia (increased irritability, fatigue, and depersonalisation); to some symptoms of psychosis, like abnormal organ sensation, to cenesthopathy (Kenyon, 1966). Hypochondria has been associated with the elusiveness of perceived symptoms and has, therefore, been linked to concepts of hysteria, depression, psychosis, neurosis, and health anxiety for millennia. Hypochondria cannot be described as a standalone medical condition because it lacks a clear causal basis, making it challenging to identify the cause of the symptoms.

Debates about medically unexplained symptoms have persisted in medicine and psychology, with various theories and their respective refutations (Crampton, 2024; Vermeir et al., 2021). Still, the dilemmas have never ceased, and patients suffering from unexplained symptoms have often not been taken seriously. The uncertain attitude is also evident in the changes in the diagnostic classification. In 2013, the *Diagnostic and Statistical Manual of Mental Disorders* (DSM-5) replaced it with new categories such as somatic symptom disorder and illness anxiety disorder (American Psychiatric Association, 2013). However, removing hypochondriasis from the DSM-5 has increased confusion about naming and diagnosis. One reason for this confusion is that hypochondriasis remained an official diagnostic category in the 11th Revision of the International Classification of Diseases (ICD-11), where it overlaps with obsessive-compulsive and anxiety disorders and is classified alongside health anxiety disorder (van den Heuvel et al., 2014; World Health Organization, 2019). Unfortunately, these medical labels primarily categorise the issues without addressing patients' fears or the frustration experienced by clinicians. Changing the labels did not solve the problem of medically unexplained symptoms. Instead, it led patients to seek their explanations for their symptoms, often turning to the internet for answers. The medical classification of hypochondria has also been challenging and controversial because, for people who suffer from medically unexplained symptoms, the problem is not just the physical symptoms themselves but what these symptoms may mean to the individual and the frustration and anxiety associated with them (Lane, 2024a). Hypochondria and health anxiety are, therefore, also a problem of meaning-making, a kind of hermeneutics. One could say that these individuals are hypersensitive readers of the texts of their bodies (Belling, 2006). In a qualitative meta-summary of studies about lived experiences of people with medically unexplained symptoms, eight typical themes were found: the need to feel understood, struggling with isolation, 'sense of self' in strain, facing uncertainty, searching for explanations, ambivalence about diagnosis, disappointed by healthcare, and active coping (Polakovská & Řiháček, 2022). The eight themes represent the main psychological and social issues adults and adolescents face when struggling with medically unexplained symptoms.

Although traditionally associated primarily with medically unexplained symptoms, health and illness anxiety does not solely pertain to individuals who lack a definable illness; it also encompasses the uncertainties arising from patients' doubts about their doctors. In this sense, it can be seen as the Achilles' heel of medicine, pointing to the uncertainty of diagnosis and the frustration that scientific progress does not yield the expected results. As Belling (2012) stated, hypochondria and related concepts can be viewed as a sceptical response to societal expectations of expertise and scientific progress. Perhaps this position of disbelief and frustration is also one of the reasons why the person who is overly concerned about illness is often portrayed as a ridiculous figure. A classic literary example of this, which has had a significant impact on public thinking and discourse on the subject, is *Molière*'s play *The Imaginary Invalid* (*The Hypochondriac*). In it, the patient Argan, learning partly from his own experience, eventually becomes a doctor himself, thus merging the figures of doctor and patient and their mutual doubt (Belling, 2012). It is exciting to note that in one of Molière's contemporary performances, he himself, playing the role of Argan, coughed up blood, and the audience was unsure whether this was an act or reality. Molière, incidentally, had tuberculosis, and this incident also shows that the label hypochondria does not mean that one cannot have a detectable disease. As hypochondria is often associated with medically unexplained symptoms, this label tends to categorise clients with these symptoms as delusional, unjustifiably complaining, and mentally ill, serving to obscure the uncertainties inherent in science.

The persistence of hypochondria in the popular imagination has been aided by the fact that many scientists and artists are known to have suffered from severe health anxieties, from Charles Darwin to Marcel Proust and from Andy Warhol to Woody Allen (Baur, 1989). It has been suggested in academic discourse that hypochondria may even facilitate creativity (Belling, 2012; Heath, 2011). This also demonstrates the ambivalence surrounding the phenomenon and the especially sceptical stance of the hypochondriac. A good example is Woody Allen, whose work makes it difficult to determine whether it focuses on the attributes of a fictional character when he portrays different manifestations of health anxiety or on his traits. In a 'self-revelatory' article in *The New York Times*, he wrote:

> I don't experience imaginary maladies – my maladies are real. What distinguishes my hysteria is that at the appearance of the mildest symptom, let's say chapped lips, I instantly leap to the conclusion that the chapped lips indicate a brain tumor. Or maybe lung cancer.
>
> *(Allen, 2013)*

Writing in an ironic tone, Allen caricatures not only his own perceived or actual hypochondria and the health anxieties of contemporary society but also the trends of 'psy-culture', which schematically applies psychological theories such as the model of the stages of grief (denial, anger, bargaining, depression, acceptance):

> In the emergency room where my wife tried to talk me down, I was making my way through the five stages of grief and was up to either 'denial' or 'bargaining' when a young resident fixed me with a rather supercilious eye and said sarcastically, 'Your hickey is benign.'
>
> *(Allen, 2013)*

So, ambivalence about medically unexplained symptoms and health anxiety persists, both in professional and lay public consciousness. However, the abolition of the medical diagnostic category of hypochondriasis (and hysteria) from the DSM and the introduction of the broader concepts of health and illness anxiety also meant the democratisation of health worries. After all, worrying about one's health is a legitimate concern, even if one is supposedly perfectly healthy or at least has no detectable illness. It should also be noted that anxiety can be associated with illness in several ways, both as a consequence and as an aetiological factor (Brady & Braz, 2023; Lane, 2024a; Kellner, 1987). The latter was confirmed, for example, by a Norwegian study that received considerable media attention and found that health anxiety increased the incidence of ischaemic heart disease by 70% (Berge et al., 2016). Physical inactivity and smoking were hypothesised as mediating variables, both related to anxiety. Health anxiety can also be associated with a pre-existing condition. For example, some studies have found increased health anxiety in one-third of cancer patients; in general, however, it is up to 8.5% in chronic patients (Grassi et al., 2015; Lebel et al., 2020). These findings also point to the need to address the issue of health anxiety from both minimising and pathologising perspectives and to consider it broadly as a general determinant of health behaviour.

The many faces of health anxiety

The reason why health anxiety (and hypochondria, hysteria) has puzzled us for millennia and why this challenge remains unresolved today is that it is a textbook case of a complicated interplay of bio-psycho-socio-cultural mechanisms. In terms of psychological processes, health anxiety is the result of a variety of factors that lead to different beliefs, perceptions, and attitudes that have a significant impact on health behaviour and the development of new fears. Dysfunctional beliefs and stronger avoidance tendencies play a familiar role in the development and worsening of health anxiety (Abramowitz & Braddock, 2011; Benke et al., 2024). This can lead to overestimating the threat, assuming a higher disease incidence, and exaggerating the ease of disease transmission and severity. Another characteristic is a low tolerance for uncertainty, driven by a strong desire for complete certainty that there will be no negative consequences. Some individuals hold a rigid view, believing that being healthy means being completely symptom-free and that all physical signs and symptoms have a medical explanation, and emotional states have perfectly natural physical concomitants. Many people believe that being sick increases the risk of developing other illnesses. This belief may be linked to the psychodynamic concept that individuals with elevated levels of health anxiety possess an 'underdeveloped ego', which obstructs their ability to form a coherent body image (McDougall, 1989). Their unfulfilled needs frequently shape their body image and can be imbued with magical and superstitious beliefs. For instance, an individual may view a particular area of their body as a source of power. If they suffer from knee or ankle pain, they might become anxious or use the excuse that they are unable to perform because 'they are not on their feet'.

The sociological perspective of health anxiety suggests that disadvantaged and marginalised groups in society often lack physical security, love, and other essential resources, both from external sources and within themselves in the form of self-esteem (Barbek et al., 2022b). These groups often lack the resources, coping strategies, social support, and material means to address this deficiency. Due to the stigma surrounding mental disorders, both those affected and society often manifest and interpret psychosocial issues as more socially acceptable physical symptoms or unexplained psychosomatic illnesses.

The relationship between parents and children, along with family dynamics, is often viewed as a key factor in health anxiety (Baur, 1989; Thorgaard et al., 2018). Between the two world wars, several classic studies were conducted on adults and children who were labelled as hypochondriacs. These studies often followed participants for several years or even longer, sometimes up to a decade (Richards, 1941). Researchers found few personality differences among the participants. Still, they agreed that individuals showing signs of health anxiety typically had one or more chronic complainers in their childhood or faced an overprotective parent who labelled and medicalised their complaints. Most often, the mother was described as both 'nagging and demanding' and the abusive parent, partly due to misogyny and partly because fathers were absent in their caregiving role. Later research from the 1960s onwards shifted the blame away from mothers, as it was found that several other factors (gender differences, age, birth order), in addition to their 'pathogenic' role, clouded the picture (Thorgaard, 2017). Recent research highlights the role of cross-generational influences and indicates a positive correlation between children's health anxiety and somatosensory enhancement and these characteristics in their parents, which are significantly influenced by parents' health beliefs (Rask et al., 2024). Many parents feel anxious and insecure, which can hinder their parenting. This can cause children to constantly seek external reinforcement, leading to addictions or psychosomatic symptoms when support is absent. They may use alcohol or other addictions to cope with missing support and reduce anxiety (McDougall, 1989).

The connection between health anxiety and overall performance is significant because physical and mental well-being have become key indicators of success in our society. This is evident on social media, where health and fitness are viewed as symbols of achievement and status. Well-being comprises two aspects: observable health behaviours and both physical and mental states, as well as internal feelings of anxiety and unspoken symptoms. How individuals present these elements is influenced by personal, social, and cultural factors. This may also help explain why disadvantaged, marginalised, and migrant groups exhibit poorer health behaviours and have a higher prevalence of unexplained symptoms and health anxiety (Barbek et al., 2022a, 2022b). Individuals from these social groups with specific medical conditions may face challenges in being taken seriously by healthcare professionals. They may be labelled as overly complaining and prescribed medication for anxiety or mood disorders instead of receiving appropriate treatment. Individuals with higher social status are more likely to receive psychotherapy and support (Niemeyer & Knaevelsrud, 2023).

The perception of symptoms that are considered acceptable and even fashionable can change over time and across different cultures. For instance, in the past, it was common for people to take indigestion pills after eating heavy food. However, heavy food consumption today is less accepted, resulting in fewer complaints about related conditions such as gallstones. As for the cultural determinants of medically unexplained symptoms, it is well known that the research of the anthropologist Arthur Kleinman (1977) has shown, among other things, that while there used to be a significant difference between Chinese and Western individuals in the physical expression of depressive symptoms, this difference is now disappearing due to globalisation (Yeung et al., 2021). In the 1970s, Chinese people had higher rates of medically unexplained physical symptoms than Americans, for example, because depression was more stigmatised in Chinese culture. This difference was common to Chinese people living in China and the United States at that time. Traditionally, the most substantial stigma in China was that people with mental health problems were considered unfit for marriage. When the American Chinese community was asked about the socially unpleasant effects of depression, anxiety, and somatoform disorders, 84.5% found depression socially unpleasant, 81.1% found anxiety unpleasant, and only 55.2% found somatoform disorders with physical symptoms socially unpleasant (Kleinman, 1987). With globalisation, these differences have begun to narrow, although they still exist. For example, one study found that Koreans used more somatic terms to describe stress than Americans (Eunsoo et al., 2016).

In most cultures, expressing stress in terms of physical symptoms is the norm – people are more likely to complain about headaches or shoulder pains than to talk about their conflicts or emotional difficulties. The predominance of physical symptoms over psychological ones in doctors' surgeries is, therefore, also due to people's tendency to report 'socially acceptable' symptoms to others. This may also explain the high prevalence of medically unexplained symptoms worldwide. Interestingly, symptom presentation and explanations can vary even within Western societies. According to a study, for example, in North America, patients were more likely to explain their medically unexplained symptoms by viruses, environmental hazards, or chemical sensitivities (Bagayogo et al., 2013). In Germany, poor circulation, low blood pressure, or heart failure were found to be somewhat more common explanations. In contrast, in the UK, bowel problems were more commonly cited by patients, while in France, biliary problems were more commonly cited. However, it is essential to note that when this survey was conducted, the internet and social networking sites were less widespread, and globalisation was not as intense as today. A recent online survey of over 73,000 participants from 39 countries found that gastrointestinal symptoms and skin problems are now widely prevalent. Specifically, 40.3% of respondents reported experiencing at least one gastrointestinal symptom (Sperber et al., 2021). This raises the question of the potential impact of increased online access to health information and the growing influence of social media on these health trends.

Consulting Dr. Google: a cure or cause for health anxiety?

In recent decades, there has been a significant increase in research on online health information-seeking behaviour (OHISB), driven by both a surge in the amount of information available and the rise of shared decision-making in healthcare as opposed to previous authoritarian forms (Bratland et al., 2024). Contributing to the increased interest in research have been awareness-raising surveys such as the Australian survey in which 60% of respondents said that after searching for information about their health online, they thought they must have an illness, and 38% believed outright that their illness was fatal (Medical Director, 2019). A few years ago, a Microsoft survey noted that a basic keyword search for 'headache' is just as likely to yield results related to brain tumours as it is to caffeine withdrawal for headaches (Markoff, 2008). This can lead to serious (and incorrect) diagnoses. Yet, we insist on 'Dr Google': a survey in the UK, for example, found that the 68 million people in Britain turned to the internet for health information more than 100 million times in 1 year (BenendenHealth, 2023). The data indicate that nearly everyone searches the internet for health information about 1.5 times a year on average, and this number is increasing. In a previous survey, a quarter of the respondents reported searching for health information online several times a day (Maon et al., 2017). Furthermore, a recent analysis that tracked user-centred internet data without relying on self-reporting revealed that two-thirds of participants sought health information on the internet at least once during the three-month study period (Bachl et al., 2024).

The first survey on this topic was conducted in 2002 and found that of Americans online, 80% had searched the internet for health-related information (Renahy & Chauvin, 2006). Similarly, in Germany, 50% of internet users searched Google for health-related information in the same year. By 2010, 88% of U.S. respondents had searched for health-related information online, and a third said they did so frequently. The proportion was particularly high among women and those with a better education, including in China (Taylor, 2010; Xiong et al., 2021). According to a Eurostat survey in 2022, 52% of the population in 27 European countries used the internet regularly, not just occasionally, to look for health-related information (Eurostat, 2022). It is particularly noteworthy, and not necessarily reassuring, that at least half the users had already 'diagnosed' themselves using Google.

In recent years, several studies have addressed the beneficial and detrimental effects of using the internet to access health information, particularly concerning anxiety (Starcevic & Berle, 2015; Starcevic & Noyes, 2014; White & Horvitz, 2009b). The relationship between internet search frequency and anxiety varies among individuals, however. Often, anxiety triggers searches, which can lead to more anxiety and, in turn, more searches. No matter the cause, conducting online searches is frequently linked to higher levels of health anxiety compared to anxiety levels before the search (Starcevic, 2017). These findings have given rise to the concept of *cyberchondria* (White & Horvitz, 2009a). Like hypochondria, cyberchondria involves problematic, sometimes addictive behaviour and is associated with increased health anxiety. Cyberchondria is the excessive search for medical or health information on the internet. It is characterised by a compulsive, irresistible urge to search for self-assurance. The initial relief, if any, is usually short-lived, but the anxiety and distress intensify during the search and continue. Online search becomes dominant in a person's life, taking precedence over other interests or daily activities, even though the search may have negative consequences. A systematic analysis of 61 studies found that although cyberchondriac behaviour is intended to be reassuring, in many cases, it leads to increased anxiety, stress, and other negative consequences (Vismara et al., 2020).

Cyberchondria is not considered a disease and is not a separate diagnostic category. It is distinguished from severe health anxiety by the typical behavioural pattern (i.e. the amount and quality of time spent online). This behaviour is reinforced and exacerbated by beliefs like 'everything is there on the internet', so it is not worth stopping the search. However, once an addiction develops, it cannot be easily stopped. Searching itself also becomes an anxiety-reducing tool after a while, creating a self-perpetuating cycle. A qualitative study examining the lived experiences of cyberchondria revealed that participants aimed to comprehend their issues and determine resolution strategies, gain reassurance by having 'done something' regarding their problems, or connect with others who faced similar challenges (McManus et al., 2015). In order to better identify the different behavioural components of cyberchondria and its potentially harmful effects, a multidimensional measure, the Cyberchondria Severity Scale (McElroy & Shevlin, 2014), was developed, which includes the following factors: *compulsion* (the involuntary nature of health-related searches), *distress* (negative emotional states and physical reactions associated with the search), *excessiveness and reassurance-seeking* (seeking reassurance from a professional), and *mistrust of professionals* (conflict over whether to trust a doctor or information on the internet). As there is no universally accepted definition, measuring the prevalence of cyberchondria is very challenging. However, studies suggest that cyberchondria – or the pattern of behaviour that the available questionnaire can measure – is associated with several psychological variables. First, low self-esteem is a determinant, but this does not influence the development of the problem per se, but through the pre-existing health anxiety and obsessive-compulsive symptoms (Bajcar & Babiak, 2021). Another typical influencing factor is the fear of anxiety and the belief that anxiety leads to severe physical and mental symptoms. Another factor is pain catastrophising, characterised by excessive worry about pain and exaggerating its severity. Finally, the development of cyberchondria is influenced by metacognitive beliefs, characterised by distorted thinking, the fear that the idea of the disease will bring about the disease, and superstitious beliefs and rituals aimed at preventing the disease. However, as the definition of cyberchondria itself is not well defined, these links are not strong. Likely, cyberchondria is primarily driven by an intolerance of uncertainty and ambiguity, as well as doubts about the reliability of sources (Starcevic, 2023). Therefore, strengthening trust in institutions, experts, researchers, and health professionals is an important goal. In this respect, the COVID-19 pandemic served as a 'global case study' and highlighted the contradictions in the concept of cyberchondria.

During the coronavirus pandemic, there was a rise in problematic internet use, including internet gambling, pornography, and general internet addiction (Király et al., 2020). Health anxiety and increased health-related internet searches also became prominent, with media outlets like *Elle* magazine featuring a journalist who 'diagnosed' herself with cyberchondria (Hirschlag, 2020). Scientific interest in the connection between internet searches and health anxiety has also increased (Jungmann & Witthöft, 2020). Some researchers have found that individuals who felt well informed about the coronavirus and had better emotional regulation skills exhibited less anxiety and less compulsive internet searching. However, established 'viral anxiety' increased cyberchondria (Jungmann et al., 2024). Other researchers have also found that some personality traits – irritability, anxiety, worry, resentment, sadness, and low self-esteem – may have amplified health anxiety and increased internet searching during COVID-19. They also noted this was more pronounced in women (Maftei & Holman, 2020). However, this result may also stem from the fact that women are significantly more likely to voice their concerns, and societies still label health-related issues as a 'women's issue'. Research on adolescents emphasised the impact of age and family influences, revealing that those whose parents faced greater challenges with digital technology and experienced increased stress during the COVID-19 pandemic exhibited higher levels of anxiety (Akgül & Ergin, 2020; Liu et al., 2022). Although differences were found in the manifestations of cyberchondria, the correlation was also reversed: higher levels of compulsive internet searching and health anxiety in adolescent children were also predictive of higher levels of stress in their parents. Starcevic et al. (2020) summarised the characteristics observed during the COVID-19 pandemic in a model and also proposed remedies for the problem behaviours described in each dimension. They highlighted the difficulties of coping with uncertainty, questioning the reliability of online information, struggles with information overload, and ineffective online reassurance-seeking. Although the model was developed in response to the coronavirus pandemic, its components, explanations, and coping strategies can be applied to other issues and situations. Therefore, it could be seen as a general guideline for understanding and addressing the links between health anxiety and problematic internet use. However, several unresolved questions and contradictions remain regarding the concept of cyberchondria. Considering the studies reviewed above through a critical lens, they were conducted in relatively affluent nations with easy access to the internet. Much of the data is self-reported, which introduces various limitations, and the studies lack contextual relevance.

Reconsidering cyberchondria

Although the concept of cyberchondria has yielded promising results quickly, it has also faced significant criticism that must be considered. Thomas (2023) described the problematic nature of cyberchondria in that it is virtually limited to one measure, the Cyberchondria Severity Scale, and has been predominantly assessed in students. Studies like measures of behavioural addiction confirm this, but rather relate to factors of anxiety (Mestre-Bach & Potenza, 2023). Recent studies have also questioned the specificity of cyberchondria related to illness anxiety (Jungmann et al., 2024).

Similarly, there is no consensus on whether cyberchondria should be managed along the lines of anxiety, obsessive-compulsive-related disorders (OCRDs), or behavioural addictions. Brown et al. (2019) openly argued that there is no need for a definition of cyberchondria, but that it is sufficient to use the category of 'online health research' (OHR) instead and examine its relationship with health anxiety. Research indicates that OHR can empower individuals and reduce anxiety; however, it may also have alarming consequences, leading to distress or compulsive behaviour (Starcevic, 2020). Therefore, a unified explanatory model of OHR should be considered to distinguish between problematic and compulsive OHR and highlight the role of underlying positive and negative metacognitions. This line of thought was continued by Schimmenti (2023), who drew attention to the stigmatising concept of cyberchondria, which positions the user as a passive sufferer. They propose a motivational framework for understanding problematic internet use, which they argue can help understand the roles and purposes of online behaviour. This would avoid oversimplifying explanations, labelling, and pathologising dysfunctional internet-use behaviour as an addiction. This would also allow us to better understand the experiences of users in the internet environment and their health anxiety patterns and thus open opportunities for prevention. We might also consider that it is not only the individual's anxiety that can facilitate the escalation of anxiety-provoking content but also the algorithms of internet search engines (Elliott, 2024).

Starcevic (2023) suggested that while uncertainties around the concept persist, attention should be directed towards preventing problematic online health searches until theoretical issues are resolved. He highlighted the role of health literacy, pointing out that higher health literacy is associated with lower cyberchondria. The first step in prevention should be to inform users about what they can expect from the internet, so that they do not have unrealistic expectations about the explanations they can receive for illnesses. The next step, he wrote, was to educate users about information overload and how too much conflicting information can often cause people to lose control and stop looking for clear evidence. He then emphasised the importance of managing uncertainty and developing users' abilities to recognise and tolerate ambiguity, a crucial feature of constructive online information-seeking. Finally, he pointed to the need to help users distinguish between reliable and unreliable sources.

Reducing anxiety through health empowerment

Considering the information above, many questions remain about the connection between health anxiety and increased internet use and how online resources might be able to help reduce health anxiety. A review study revealed that although health anxiety rose from 1985 to 2017, this rise could not be directly associated with the increase in internet use (Kosic et al., 2020). The study's subjects were all students. Members of *Generation Z* (those born between 1995 and 2010), who are digital natives, tend to rely on the internet for getting health-related information at much higher rates than previous generations. However, some studies have found that they have the lowest rates of health empowerment (Jiao et al., 2023). This is likely because people in this age group generally experience fewer health problems; still, we should prioritise establishing preventive health education and health awareness at this age. From this perspective, the development of health empowerment is crucial. The good news for this generation is that they are the most digitally literate. However, with their increased digital presence, it is crucial to be aware of the risk of problematic internet use and the prevention of health anxiety, which is where health empowerment can help.

The issue of digital health literacy also raises questions of equity and autonomy, some of which are generational and some sociodemographic. The development of digital health will enhance access to digital services and other resources for individuals with limited financial means. In turn, it will also provide opportunities for high-resource individuals, the 'worried well', to manage more health problems independently, freeing up time and provider capacity for those who have difficulty accessing healthcare and who have previously been difficult to reach and support (Nickel et al., 2023). Research into and development of levels of motivation and health empowerment are also of particular importance here, as is the fact that while it is hoped that digital health literacy will increase among young people and thus reduce health anxiety, the number of older people living with chronic illness and dementia will increase due to increased life expectancy. From the perspective of cyberchondria and health anxiety prevention in general and the promotion of good health behaviours specifically, it should also be noted that health empowerment and adequate information need to be present at the same time as empowered, active, but ill-informed individuals can experience serious negative consequences (Mohammadinia et al., 2024; Schulz & Nakamoto, 2022). An example of this is the case of vaccine sceptics during the COVID-19 pandemic, where health worries about the effects of the vaccine were greater than fears about the consequences of contracting the virus.

In addition to developing health literacy, recent research has highlighted the importance of emotion regulation, indicating it as a significant mediating factor between health anxiety and cyberchondria (Fang & Mustaque, 2024; Nasiri et al., 2023). Similarly, health literacy has appeared to moderate the relationship between health anxiety and emotion regulation and health-promoting behaviours between emotion regulation and cyberchondria. We can, therefore, see that this is a very complex set of relationships; consequently, neither the theoretical concept nor the prevention and treatment strategies can be simplified to a one-dimensional behavioural addiction model, such as cyberchondria. A complex approach is fundamental because some research suggests that even health professionals' health literacy is not always perfect, and they can also have cyberchondria (Raziye et al., 2022). One of the reasons why doctors are reluctant to deal with patients with excessive health anxiety is that they are confronted with their own, mostly repressed, 'hypochondriac' anxiety, which stems from the fact that they are constantly faced with the fragility of life in the course of their work (Groopman, 2003).

One way forward might be to consider how to assist potential patients on the same platform, rather than labelling people who search the internet for information about their condition as 'cyberchondriacs' (Leykin et al., 2012). Presumably, users are looking for these options, and we know that most of them – 63% on average – consider the information they find on the internet reliable (IPSOS, 2022). It is, therefore, very important to help people evaluate sources and increase their access to professionally validated, reliable information, as well as support tools and care (Meskó, 2020). This highlights the importance of reconsidering individual, community, and social responsibility. Although health anxiety has become a common topic in public discussions, the media and internet often portray health as an individual concern rather than a shared responsibility within communities or societies at large (Lewis, 2006). This portrayal can lead to concerns about meeting sociocultural expectations, especially when these expectations are not clearly communicated and instead remain concealed or are challenging to comprehend. Self-management has become a significant topic in health communication, as it is crucial for maintaining health and promoting recovery. Recognising that not everyone has the means to prioritise self-care is essential. Public communication often assumes that everyone has equal freedom of choice and autonomy; however, this is not always the case, as various psychosocial and cultural factors influence it.

Thus, how can we ensure that everyone is well informed about their health in a way that does not increase their anxiety but improves their physical and mental well-being? Naturally, there are significant differences in users' needs, digital health literacy, social and cultural backgrounds, health status, and many other factors. People also seek a wide range of content and have various reasons for seeking information. It is challenging to determine the impact of these searches on the users and those for or with whom they are searching. It is common for a user to search for someone who cannot use the internet or may be unwilling to address their condition. Additionally, the internet facilitates the creation of communities where people share experiences of health conditions, post helpful information, and form support groups (Ngenye & Wright, 2022). Furthermore, some health-related communication occurs through email and messaging. The role of the internet in building communities is as important as it is in addressing the problems of individuals who seek information in a solitary, obsessive, and anxious manner.

Again, we must return to questions of definition and the extent to which the medicalised concept of cyberchondria reflects the medical profession's fear of losing its monopoly on knowledge and the extent to which it can be a pathology. In 1998, with the advent of the internet, the *British Medical Journal* published the question of whether we are witnessing the onset of an epidemic of misinformation (Coiera, 1998). The entire internet was portrayed in this article and elsewhere as a dangerous space. In this view, the layperson is not an autonomous, independent user or consumer of health products but a potential victim often misled by medical pseudo-information, encouraged to engage in unhealthy behaviour, and driven to develop compulsive addictions. This view is still held today, even though internet use has become an integral part of everyday life and a primary arena for managing health information. Fortunately, the question of how to ensure the quality of health and medical information on the internet is now getting more attention. This raises numerous professional and ethical concerns; however, information control may also present a barrier to self-organised support groups. Conversely, discussions about 'quality' are often framed within a giver-receiver model, where the professional 'gives' information and the lay recipient passively 'receives' it. This approach overlooks the interactive nature of the internet, where users are not only recipients but also active creators and shapers of content. The empowering, proactive, and collaborative approach should be strengthened. Support programmes, interventions, and platforms should be created where users can safely rely on posted information and thus reduce their health anxiety.

Conclusion

The perception of health anxiety among laypeople and professionals has evolved considerably over time and has become heavily medicalised due to various scientific, social, and cultural influences. Throughout different periods in medical history, defining health anxiety has posed significant challenges, mainly because of shifting diagnostic terminology and uncertainty, as well as biased and gendered views related to 'hypochondria' and medically unexplained symptoms. Today, the emergence of the term 'cyberchondria', linked to the rise of the internet, highlights the adverse effects of seeking health information online, such as increased anxiety and dependency. However, there is also evidence suggesting that the internet can effectively empower individuals by enhancing health knowledge and digital health literacy. Developing various forms of health literacy, especially digital health literacy, can help reduce anxiety and foster health empowerment. Users do not merely consume content; they actively create and influence it. They can share personal experiences and healthcare insights, which are invaluable for conditions often overlooked by healthcare professionals. Consequently, the internet's role in building communities is as important as its capacity to help individuals find information more confidently and with less anxiety. While this raises concerns about the behaviour of these individuals, it can also be viewed as a proactive approach that may alleviate the burden on overwhelmed healthcare systems.

4

PSYCHOSOCIAL CHALLENGES OF MONITORING THE ANXIOUS BODY

A few decades ago, it might have seemed futuristic to consider that 'How are you?' would one day be supplanted by 'What does your data show?' as an introduction to a conversation. Today, however, it is easy to envision checking our smartwatches and accessing all our data and reports at our fingertips. As of 2024, more than 454 million individuals globally are using wearable devices to monitor their health, and market forecasts indicate that this number will continue to grow rapidly (Statista Research Department, 2024). According to some statistics, 23% of men and 21.8% of women worldwide already own a smartwatch (Shewale, 2024). Additionally, many people use self-tracking methods to measure and record various bodily functions and health parameters. The tradition of monitoring and recording our health and personal experiences is not new; it dates back centuries through diaries, albums, and other offline methods (Humphreys, 2018). However, the rise of the information society and the advancement of digitalisation have ushered in a new era. In recent years, an increasing number of social scientists have begun to explore the implications of this trend on health behaviours, our relationships with ourselves and others, and the potential effects on future generations.

Tracked bodies in the 'age of anxiety'

With the advancement of digital technology, the continuous monitoring of behaviour and bodily functions has become so prevalent that 'self-tracking' was added as a separate entry in the Oxford English Dictionary in 2015, entering the international public domain (Oxford Dictionaries, 2015). While self-tracking originally referred to monitoring and collecting data based on individual fitness and health goals, recent observations indicate that it is increasingly evolving into a

DOI: 10.4324/9781003517788-4

social phenomenon characterised by complex interaction patterns and varying expectations. While this can be motivating for many users, it can also lead to feelings of anxiety (Feng et al., 2021). Deborah Lupton (2016, 2018), a leading expert in the field, has demonstrated that the increasing demand for digital data usage has emerged at commercial, corporate, and governmental levels. This trend raises broader issues related to biopolitics, citizenship, and identity. Lupton (2016) identifies five modes of self-tracking: private, communal, pushed, imposed, and exploited. She highlights the complex interpersonal and sociopolitical contexts surrounding these modes and their implications for control, power, and surveillance.

While many people use digital self-tracking tools and a growing amount of analysis exists on the topic, significant uncertainty persists about the use of these devices. Factors beyond individual motivations often influence self-tracking, which adds to this uncertainty. This can have serious consequences for relationships with others and oneself, particularly regarding body image and self-image (Boldi & Rapp, 2022). Most bodily functions are not directly accessible and can only be measured using various instruments and diagnostic tools, which means they are not part of our immediate experience of our bodies and selves. This raises an important question: can the entirety of body and mind functioning be accurately captured in a quantified form, and can self-monitoring truly be fully realised?

The first conference on 'body-wearable computers' or body-sensing devices was held in 1997 (Lupton, 2016). At that time, the focus was primarily on detecting internal processes and emotional experiences in workplaces or during artistic creation. However, since the early 2000s, the development of smartwatches has significantly advanced the practice of self-monitoring. The Quantified Self (QS) movement, which promotes self-tracking internationally, originated in California's Silicon Valley in 2007 (Wolf, 2016). It was primarily driven by white, middle-class American men working in the tech industry. Members of this movement argued that the ancient maxim 'know thyself' could be achieved through measurement and quantification (Wolf, 2009).

Several studies have confirmed that self-tracking can enhance physical and psychological self-awareness (Li et al., 2021). Many users report positive outcomes such as improved health and greater awareness of themselves and their environment. Studies have shown that self-tracking devices can increase the awareness of one's body and behaviours (Feng et al., 2021). In many cases, lasting behavioural changes persist after self-monitoring has stopped (Lupton, 2014). However, researchers have also highlighted the downsides: users track too much information at once, struggle to process it, fail to identify their symptoms correctly, and develop a sense of fatigue with tracking (Ajana, 2020; Choe et al., 2014). Much also depends on the self-tracker's general mindset and attitude towards monitoring, which is a key determinant of personal experience (Hancı et al., 2021). This may also contribute to the fact that for some people, self-tracking provides a sense of control over their health, well-being and productivity, and the benefits of personalised healthcare, while others feel it points to their weaknesses and lack of discipline and, therefore, emphasise the disciplining, disempowering effects of self-tracking (Dennison et al., 2013; Sharon, 2017). Many people also fear that the tools will control them, that is influence their behaviour uncontrollably, create dependencies, and even lead to personality or identity changes (Wieczorek et al., 2022).

Critics argue that the objectivity of numerical values is debatable, even though they are often presented as neutral and impartial. Individual perspectives, subjective experiences, and sociocultural influences inevitably affect interpretation, and quantification inherently involves simplification (Sharon, 2017). The sociopolitical context, value judgements, and scientific biases shape the algorithms that record and analyse measurement results. In the context of self-tracking, this suggests that categories such as well-being, health, and happiness are often translated into specific ideal values. These values tend to reflect normative stereotypes and may pressure users to adjust their behaviour to meet these standards (Dorfmann et al., 2023). This can lead to a limited way of experiencing life, which may alienate individuals from their authentic experiences, knowledge, and intuition based on bodily sensations. As a result, feelings of insecurity and anxiety can increase significantly. One limitation of research on the effectiveness of wearable devices is that it is primarily conducted in high-resource settings, leading to a socioculturally biased perspective. Furthermore, this research tends to focus more on monitoring physical health rather than addressing mental health issues (Huhn et al., 2022). However, an intriguing study analysing a large corpus of 8 million books using Google Ngram reveals a significant increase over the past 50 years in the co-occurrence of the terms 'anxiety', 'depression', and 'digitalisation' (Teepe et al., 2023). A growing body of evidence indicates that digital technologies can effectively enhance mental healthcare, encompassing a range of interventions and artificial intelligence (AI) solutions (Bond et al., 2023; Lau et al., 2024). This focus on digital solutions is significant, as current professional capacity falls short of meeting a fraction of mental healthcare needs. For instance, in developed countries, there are approximately 9 psychiatrists for every 100,000 inhabitants, whereas in low-income regions, this number drops to just 1 psychiatrist for every 10 million inhabitants, and preventive services are equally insufficient (Ahmed et al., 2023; Khosravi et al., 2024). Therefore, digital solutions in mental health are essential, encompassing therapeutic interventions and training, education, and screening programmes. However, as discussed below, much more research is needed on their reliability and effectiveness.

Self-tracking applications can be beneficial for detecting and managing anxiety. They may help overcome issues like stigma, social desirability bias, and underdiagnosis that often accompany traditional methods (Das & Gavade, 2024). Recently, experience in the field has grown, with practitioners noting the benefits of these technologies. However, they emphasise that blended or adjunctive solutions are the safest and most effective, including in-person consultations with specialists for prevention or treatment (Bond et al., 2023). This approach helps clients avoid unverified applications, reduces misunderstandings and anxiety, and counters 'technological solutionism', where clients believe that technology solves all issues.

Experts increasingly observe that while wearable technology can reduce anxiety, it may also worsen health-related anxiety (Lane, 2024b; Meskó, 2023; Nieslanik, 2024). In particular, the constant checking and re-checking of self-tracking devices can lead to fixation, and users often do not realise until it is too late that their heightened anxiety is linked to this behaviour. Furthermore, it is essential to recognise that increased anxiety in affected individuals is not always tied to changes in physiological indicators, and users frequently do not communicate their concerns to professionals (Oostrum, 2024; Rosman et al., 2024).

Professionals emphasise the importance of developing self-regulation and stress awareness in this context. This involves users being able to monitor their quantified data while also identifying, understanding, and managing their anxiety and stress responses (González Ramirez et al., 2023). This process can be supported by advancements in smartwatches, such as heart rate variability (HRV) tracking and biofeedback solutions, which provide real-time stress feedback and personalised stress management interventions (Jerath et al., 2023). Unregulated and unprocessed negative emotions, such as anxiety and anger, are linked to the development and worsening of various diseases, particularly cardiovascular disease. Research indicates that patients experiencing specific cardiovascular symptoms, like atrial fibrillation, are more likely to monitor their condition and attribute irregular heart rhythms to stress (Cheung & Saad, 2024). This can increase stress and anxiety (Rosman et al., 2020).

Lifelogging involves maintaining a digital record of daily activities, aiding self-reflection and coping, which may reduce negative emotions (Dobbins & Fairclough, 2016). It can be enhanced by tracking body awareness, health behaviours, and lifestyle. A key issue is ensuring that recording experiences supports self-reflection without causing anxiety or health concerns. Virtual reality (VR), increasingly used in digital mental health, helps process experiences and reduce anxiety. First used decades ago for fears and phobias (May, 2024), VR is now common in mental health treatment. Research shows that VR can be quicker, more effective, and engaging than traditional methods, helping therapists identify anxiety-provoking situations and reassure clients. VR also effectively treats chronic pain, including headaches, neck, shoulder, and back pain, as well as phantom limb pain (Wong et al., 2022). This may be due to the link between chronic pain, anxiety, and depression.

Various digital solutions, including chatbots, have shown promising results in reducing anxiety and depression among patients with chronic physical conditions such as arthritis and diabetes (MacNeill et al., 2024). Chatbots are particularly effective in providing social support to disadvantaged groups, especially young people. However, it is essential to consider the special educational needs of older and less digitally literate users when introducing these newer technologies (Limpanopparat et al., 2024). A comparison of 10 chatbot applications available in the Google Play Store and the Apple App Store identified a significant risk that could impact users of all ages (Haque & Rubya, 2023). Chatbots are always available;

therefore, users might prefer them over face-to-face interactions with family and friends. This preference can lead to social isolation, making users less likely to seek help during times of crisis or distress (Herbener & Damholdt, 2025).

One of the first successful examples of AI-based treatment for health anxiety is the Otis chatbot, developed in New Zealand during the COVID-19 pandemic (Goonesekera & Donkin, 2022). Based on cognitive behavioural techniques, this intervention improved users' anxiety levels, subjective well-being, and quality of life. Other chatbots, such as Woebot and the Fido application, have also been effectively used to treat general anxiety and depression, particularly among young people. Users of these chatbots have reported a decrease in feelings of loneliness (Karkosz et al., 2024). The high demand for support in the mental health field is evident from the fact that by 2024, there were 475 chatbots with terms like 'therapist', 'therapy', 'psychologist', or 'psychiatrist' in their names (Tidy, 2024). The most popular was a bot named *Psychologist*, created by a 30-year-old user from New Zealand using the Character.ai platform. Initially developed for himself and his friends, the creator was surprised that it became the most popular chatbot providing psychological support. Within a year, it received 78 million messages, primarily relating to anxiety and depression (Tidy, 2024). Another example is the Chinese chatbot Xiaoice, which has hundreds of millions of users, with some estimates suggesting a billion (Agence France-Presse, 2021). With the rapid development of chatbots and AI mental health applications, a question arises regarding whether these technologies, which lack genuine caring abilities yet create an illusion of care, may be misleading for users (Khawaja & Bélisle-Pipon, 2023). As a result, new concepts such as 'artificial empathy' and 'artificial intimacy' have emerged (Hamrick, 2023; Turkle, 2024). These concepts highlight the necessity to reconsider issues related to self and identity.

Wearable tech, fluid identities

It is now widely recognised that we live in an era of continuous self-transformation, which includes the renewal and development of both the body and mind (Rose, 1998). This phenomenon is closely connected to practices and cultural expectations surrounding self-realisation, personal growth, health promotion, nutrition, and fitness. Furthermore, constant self-monitoring has become a social norm, particularly in Western countries. Technological advancements have emerged as a key issue of how people interact with non-human actors in various social networks, and how this affects their self-experiences and identity formation (Latour, 2005). Digital devices are increasingly been seen as extensions of our bodies and identities, becoming agents of action in their own right, as they serve as the means through which we navigate our surroundings and express ourselves. Technologies are integrated into our understanding of the body and the self, shaping our relationship with our physical existence, interactions, choices, and environments. Instead of merely inducing anxiety, the constant feedback and visualisation of data can encourage us to connect with our bodies and become attuned to their needs. Over time, individuals may internalise the practice of self-monitoring, developing an awareness that promotes new behaviour patterns, which could make the technology unnecessary (Kristensen & Prigge, 2018). However, it can also lead individuals to become overly dependent on self-monitoring, resulting in having anxiety about their bodies and health, as well as a compulsive fixation on monitoring their behaviours (Nickel et al., 2023).

Today, data collected through apps or other platforms becomes, or at least appears to become, expert knowledge (Prior, 2003). The body-self created through self-monitoring is both the subject and the product of measurement and interpretation. However, self-tracking is about measuring and extending the self, even creating a kind of 'exoself'. Indeed, inherent in self-tracking is the potential to create a narrative that reinforces the self, constructed from data that supports self-identity (Sharon, 2017). Representatives of the QS movement emphasise that individual self-monitoring projects can serve as platforms for establishing independent identities and experiencing personal autonomy (Wolf, 2016). They contend that body sensing and self-tracking reflect a countercultural and non-conformist attitude. This is partly because digital processes facilitate immediate and widespread data sharing, allowing direct comparisons with others, unlike previous self-tracking methods such as handwritten diaries or paper spreadsheets. This phenomenon can be viewed as a form of democratisation of the self. Furthermore, this trend can be interpreted as laypeople's conscious or unconscious rebellion against expert knowledge, which can foster a sense of autonomy and empowerment. However, alternative interpretations view this movement as merely facilitating increased control and surveillance by the technology industry or, more broadly, the health industry (Chiodo, 2022; Lupton, 2012).

Autonomy can be strengthened and weakened by self-tracking devices that collect intimate information about us, effectively becoming our confidants and anthropomorphised companions (Rettberg, 2018). Many developers recognise this dynamic, which might explain why the built-in assistant Siri on iPhones is designed to have a friendly female persona. However, from a critical perspective, the prevalence of female voices in digital assistants may reflect stereotypes about gender roles and power relations. This consideration may also shed light on naming one of the first famous chatbots, as ELIZA, created by Joseph Weizenbaum in 1966. ELIZA was modelled after Rogerian empathetic psychologists yet communicated within the confines of traditional gender roles (Rettberg, 2018).

Monitoring the health of loved ones

So far, we have primarily focused on different forms of self-tracking from an individual perspective. However, monitoring practices do not occur in isolation; various interpersonal, cultural, and political influences shape them. How these practices are utilised can also impact relationships (Lomborg & Frandsen, 2016).

In the context of families and couples, co-tracking – meaning joint monitoring of fitness and health – can serve as an essential tool for providing social support and encouraging healthy behaviours. Tracking technology can assist in supporting elderly parents and monitoring children's health behaviours, fostering various forms of 'digital kinship' (Hjorth et al., 2020). However, this co-tracking can also lead to monitoring among family members, potentially causing tension and increasing health anxiety. Additionally, tracking changes in physical health can create specific power dynamics within the family or couple relationships. For instance, research indicates that it is not uncommon for husbands or male partners to monitor women's weight data and hold them accountable closely if they do not meet certain expectations (Will et al., 2020). The 'tracking the tracker' phenomenon occurs with various health measurements such as blood pressure, blood glucose, and calorie intake. Couples often monitor each other's measurements closely and may express concern or outrage if the results are inappropriate (Hardey, 2022). While this behaviour is typically motivated by a genuine concern for the partner's well-being, it can also create a feeling of surveillance and control, which may negatively impact the relationship and overall health behaviour. For instance, older couples often take their daily blood pressure readings simultaneously, record the data together, and refer to their measurements as 'our blood pressure'. This shared attitude may reflect a symbiotic relationship in which both partners feel connected to each other's health. Similar dynamics can be observed in couples of any age who exercise, diet, or take vitamins together to maintain their fitness and health. They frequently track their progress using self-tracking devices, apps, or traditional methods such as pen and paper.

An essential factor in a couple's relationship is the degree to which health promotion activities are a shared commitment. This includes whether they reflect a shared set of values or if one partner participates for reasons other than genuine conviction. For example, one partner may be more dominant, leading their values to take precedence. Alternatively, loyalty to each other might overshadow individual health needs, resulting in activities that are only possible as joint endeavours (Umberson et al., 2018). One partner in a couple may feel concerned about their partner's health and, as a result, may 'sacrifice' their preferences to support them. This could involve joining in on exercise routines, adhering to a diet, or engaging in self-monitoring, not out of personal motivation or enjoyment, but out of concern. Additionally, sharing health data or engaging in self-monitoring can create competition and anxiety between partners. This trend is widespread among young people, who may compare each other's data to gauge their own strength, aiming to see whose health metrics are better or 'more perfect' (Klier et al., 2022).

Discussing and tracking data about our bodies, health, and behaviours can have numerous positive benefits, often outweighing any disadvantages (Pennington & Dam, 2023). This practice not only encourages healthy habits and chronic disease management but can also enhance the bond and solidarity between couples, helping their relationship to grow and develop. While sharing this information can sometimes mask the underlying conflicts, it can also serve as a tool for addressing and resolving them in a constructive manner. These aspects are fundamental in the context of telemedicine, self-management, and anxiety.

Self-care and digital health empowerment

Home self-tracking and remote patient monitoring are vital tools for promoting health, as they enhance patients' autonomy regarding specific diseases, increase their sense of safety, and reduce health-related anxiety. Many national health governments prioritise the development of devices for these purposes, aiming to lower hospital admissions and healthcare costs (Vudathaneni et al., 2024). One notable example is diabetes management, where a detector implanted inside the patient's body continuously transmits signals to the doctor through a wireless device. This technology saves the doctor and the patient time, energy, and money. Another crucial area to focus on is promoting healthy behaviours in disadvantaged social groups through self-tracking devices. There is a common misconception that these groups have a lower affinity for digital technology; however, several studies, including a recent survey conducted among homeless individuals by a Hungarian sociological research group, reveal otherwise. They found that 69.6% of respondents own a mobile phone, and 39.9% own a smartphone. Additionally, 11.2% of participants reported using a mobile health application (Radó et al., 2022). This data suggests that we can leverage this technology to offer a variety of supportive and health-promoting interventions, considering the basic needs and context of users.

Self-tracking devices offer a vision of a future where individuals take a more active role in managing their health, generating data that can aid medical decision-making and research. However, this optimistic outlook is accompanied by several social and ethical concerns (Sharon, 2017). Most self-tracking devices are designed for general consumer use rather than specific clinical applications. For instance, among cardiac patients, tools such as heart rate monitors, sleep trackers, and step counters have proven beneficial for self-care. However, they have also led to feelings of uncertainty, fear, and anxiety in some cases (Andersen et al., 2020). Manufacturers need to verify the accuracy of their devices, minimise the occurrence of alarming and anxiety-inducing false positives, and integrate educational resources into these devices to ensure that consumers have support and guidance. Stakeholders – including technology companies, researchers, developers, healthcare professionals, patients, and healthy users – must collaborate to provide access to digital health opportunities for individuals from all backgrounds.

The good news is that self-monitoring is now achievable in many areas, making it an essential part of personalised and collaborative healthcare in more developed countries (Chén & Roberts, 2021; Lupton, 2014; Meskó et al., 2017). However, critical analysts argue that self-care is often framed in terms that cater to health-conscious, individualistic users (Wardell, 2024). They question whether this perspective risks separating health from its broader social, political, and cultural contexts. In ageing societies, for instance, there are increasingly critical concerns about what happens to older and economically disadvantaged individuals who lack digital health literacy, the ability to interpret and utilise information, or the financial means to acquire and manage health management tools (Shi et al., 2024). Other important questions arise regarding who is responsible for providing adequate information about digital health tools, how users can navigate the thousands of available apps, and how susceptible users are to the commercial interests of technology companies (Stoumpos et al., 2023; Yuen et al., 2024). Digital health advocates view the increasing availability of these tools as an opportunity to democratise healthcare, referring to it as a 'Gutenberg moment' for the industry (Topol, 2013). The authors argue that these tools are more accessible to the public than traditional text-based information, which is often paper-based and tends to cater to the educated elite – those more likely to read books than others. However, some critics question whether this increased accessibility leads to health empowerment and social justice (Hendl & Shukla, 2024).

In recent years, research has increasingly focused on how much digital health tools require users to feel empowered and how self-tracking can enhance feelings of empowerment and self-efficacy. Kapeller and Loosman (2023) suggested that while the *WHO* defines health empowerment as a process that leads to a sense of control over health-related decisions and knowledge, developers of wearable apps often place less emphasis on this processual aspect. This emphasis is crucial, as several studies analysing user experiences have explicitly identified empowerment, self-management, and personalisation as key factors driving the choice of digital health devices. Conversely, low digital health literacy and concerns about privacy are significant barriers (Madanian et al., 2023). A study investigating the relationship between empowerment and anxiety regarding digital device usage discovered that only individuals with lower openness to novelty were more likely to experience negative emotions related to wearable devices (Ryan et al., 2019). This suggests a potential link between these emotions and levels of empowerment and digital health literacy. Critical analyses raise essential questions about the role of empowerment in health promotion. Specifically, they explore to what extent empowerment as a goal truly serves individuals' autonomy needs versus meeting predetermined objectives that may reflect hidden paternalistic motives (Wieczorek et al., 2022). Additionally, we must consider whether individuals, particularly women, are being unfairly burdened with the responsibility for their health and that of their families, a responsibility that traditionally falls to the state and other institutions. This concern is highlighted by how empowerment is portrayed in health promotion discourse and advertising for self-tracking and mHealth applications, often suggesting that users already possess this empowerment. Another critical question is distinguishing between genuine empowerment, as users perceive it, and the mere illusion of empowerment created by the health promotion and commercial messaging surrounding them (Kapeller, 2024). This issue is particularly significant for applications focused on fitness or diet, as well as those that enable users to test for various health conditions or monitor diseases. In such cases, the interactive features and support built into these devices are crucial for self-management and fostering true empowerment.

In the past 15 years, the rise of self-tracking tools and social media has prompted several researchers to examine the relationship between these technologies and self-reflection (Kent, 2020; Lim, 2016; Lupton, 2012, 2016). Self-tracking often lacks introspection, and public sharing of data influences health perceptions and self-image. This can affect health behaviours, self-surveillance, and surveillance of others, leading to changes in identity. Individuals may develop a 'data self' based more on data than lived experiences, heightening uncertainty and anxiety about their body and health (Kristensen & Prigge, 2018).

This issue raises concerns about autonomy and justice, particularly regarding whether digital health empowerment truly offers disadvantaged and marginalised groups meaningful opportunities for development and improved access to health promotion (Nickel et al., 2024). Messages about digital health are often clearer to those with higher technological and health literacy. Conversely, they suggest that technology gives people significant control over their health. However, many feel disappointed and anxious about their health due to their practical experiences. Additionally, uncertainty surrounding data privacy, such as how personal information is stored and who has access to it, can evoke similar feelings of anxiety, especially among individuals with lower literacy levels (Ezeudoka & Fan, 2024). In addition to the divide between those who are able and those who are disadvantaged, it is crucial to examine the social and psychological factors that influence the use of digital health tools. Anxiety is believed to play a role as both a causal factor and a consequence, affecting further health behaviours, partly through the influence of health literacy (Fang & Mushtaque, 2024; Fitzpatrick, 2023; Sham et al., 2024; Wanger, 2024).

The dilemmas mentioned arise from the evolving definition of health, which now encompasses not only 'good' or 'bad' health but also lifestyle choices. We often feel pressured to make 'right' ethical decisions regarding self-care. The anxiety experienced by users of self-tracking tools and social media about how others will react to 'wrong' health behaviours can significantly contribute to this pressure (Riley et al., 2019). Self-tracking habits are often a proxy for body image, as people frequently share visual representations of their results on social media. Sharing lifestyle and health behaviours online also constitutes a form of self-tracking. Consequently, individual behaviour becomes heavily influenced by others as we strive to conform to the 'healthy self-images' showcased on social media, regardless of how accurately they reflect our actual conditions (Kent, 2018). In this context, physical health and lifestyle concepts are being redefined through self-monitoring and publicity. Many people are concerned that if these definitions rely solely on measurements and data, the ideas of body and health will be oversimplified. This reduction to mere numbers and images may overlook individuality and personal uniqueness, and the question of who has access to the information is also a pressing issue today.

Mindfully track your self-experience

Many current trends in self-monitoring and self-regulation – whether in therapeutic settings or everyday life – focus on experiencing bodily and psychological sensations deeply and authentically, rather than just quantifying them. A notable example is mindfulness meditation. Its digital transformations can serve as a case study for other therapeutic applications. As mindfulness has gained popularity and led to the creation of billion-dollar industries worldwide, there has been an increase in digital diaries, computer programs, and mobile apps designed to assist individuals in practising mindfulness and tracking their experiences (McGuire, 2020). This trend raises a critical question: to what extent are these tools and platforms detracting from the original essence of meditation, which focuses on monitoring direct experiences and being present in the moment?

Today, digital relaxation and meditation techniques are among the most commonly used self-monitoring methods available to the public, helping to increase body awareness and reduce stress and anxiety. Mindfulness meditation, which focuses on developing a mindful presence, has gained significant popularity over the past few decades. The global market for mindfulness meditation apps was valued at $118.8 million in 2024 and is projected to reach $218.7 million by 2030 (Research & Markets, 2025). According to Jon Kabat-Zinn (2003), the founder and leading advocate of mindfulness, it involves intentionally focusing on the present moment and experiencing it in a non-judgemental, moment-by-moment manner. The experiences of both laypeople and therapeutic professionals over the decades have shown that mindfulness – a natural, unquantifiable approach to self-monitoring and self-awareness – can be a powerful tool for overcoming stress, alleviating negative emotional states, and reducing health anxiety (Khoury et al., 2015). However, some authors have taken a critical stance on this topic, highlighting how mindfulness meditation has drifted away from its original Buddhist roots and become part of the consumer culture (Van Dame et al., 2018; Walsh, 2016). In the Western business world, mindfulness is often employed to reduce stress while keeping employees competitive and alert (Congleton et al., 2015). While meditation has clear stress-reducing benefits, emphasising the brain's universal biochemical processes and the expectation for employees to practise mindfulness raise concerns about their physical responsibility and the medicalisation of behaviour. This is especially relevant in the case of 'McMindfulness', where meditation is treated as a consumer product, stripped of its spiritual roots, and focused solely on achieving superficial relaxation and temporary adaptability (Gale, 2021; Hyland, 2015). This situation inadvertently reinforces consumer goals that go beyond individual choice, aligning more with the interests of employers or the wellness industry. Additionally, mindfulness has increasingly become entwined with digitalisation, significantly diverting the practice from its original aims and methods.

According to a major review article, by 2015, over 600 English-language mobile phone apps were promoting themselves as mindfulness meditation apps (Mani et al.,

2015). The analysis revealed that only 4% of these apps offered a genuine mindfulness programme; the majority were merely guided meditation apps or simple timers and reminders that could assist with mindfulness practice but did not encompass its full functionality. A study of 605 apps in the European market found that overall quality was relatively low, with most apps failing to meet data security and privacy standards (Schultchen et al., 2021). In addition to these conditions, genuinely effective and professionally reliable mindfulness apps support the practice through content and imagery and by incorporating ritualisation. This helps users retreat into their inner space, allowing them to return to their work or home environments feeling rejuvenated. However, very few apps meet these criteria, which explains why users often feel disappointed or misled after using apps falsely marketed as mindfulness tools. As a result, they may come to believe that mindfulness meditation and mindful presence are merely superficial or 'cheap' experiences. This is concerning, as users might apply this negative perception to other aspects of self-awareness and health monitoring. Ultimately, the dilution and commercialisation of mindfulness could detract from its original purpose, leaving stress and anxiety unresolved and steering individuals away from professionally informed support.

Mindfulness has gained widespread acceptance in the health sector, supported by extensive scientific evidence highlighting its benefits while cautioning about potential drawbacks (Macrynikola et al., 2024). Complying with the American Psychological Association app evaluation model can be very beneficial for selecting appropriate apps. The model identifies the following criteria to help mental health professionals recommend the right tool for their clients: accessibility, privacy and safety, app usability, and data integration towards the therapeutic goal (Lagan et al., 2020). However, the widely accepted, consumer-focused interpretation of mindfulness often strays from the established professional standards and scientific principles, which include radical scepticism, the need for independent peer review, and a commitment to value neutrality. This consumer-oriented approach to mindfulness is closely associated with medicalisation and heightened health consciousness (Reveley, 2016). On the one hand, mindfulness can positively teach us the importance of self-monitoring, self-care, self-management, and maintaining both physical and mental well-being from an early age. On the other hand, it can foster a mindset that insists on constant self-monitoring. This implied message indicates that you should continuously monitor your well-being, as you are never entirely well; continuous improvement of your condition is necessary. While fostering a positive sense of responsibility, this can also become an overwhelming burden if users are not equipped with the correct information, tools, and expert support to manage stress effectively and efficiently.

Unquantified selves for better health?

Socrates is believed to have claimed that an unexamined life is not worth living (Brickhouse & Smith, 1994). Paraphrasing this, the QS movement states that our experiences alone do not offer sufficient feedback for personal growth and improvement without measurement. Nonetheless, as previously discussed, a substantial internal contradiction exists within the QS movement: self-tracking can both alleviate and provoke anxiety and enhance and destabilise our sense of control (Crawley, 2022). Although the QS movement is still relatively new, counter-movements have swiftly emerged, with more individuals advocating for the advantages of unquantified lived experiences (Díaz Andrade et al., 2023). They emphasise that data from QS-tracking serves merely as raw material, which users interpret through their personal and cultural experiences. This conveys the notion of *situated objectivity* (Pantzar & Ruckenstein, 2017). Many users expect clear and straightforward results from wearable health tools, yet they frequently overlook how their expectations, perceptions, and understanding of health can influence their interpretation of the data. Consequently, many users become frustrated after a brief period and struggle to incorporate the data from these devices into their daily lives.

The development of digital self-tracking devices is ongoing and is expected to grow. Consequently, conducting further analyses and balanced evaluations is crucial while providing adequate information and expert support for the average user. This support could be enhanced by employing health information counsellors or digital health advisors with interdisciplinary training in health management, digital technologies, data privacy, medical and legal issues, and interpersonal communication (Fiske et al., 2019). Such expertise can help health professionals and everyday users maximise the benefits of these technologies while mitigating potential adverse effects.

Conclusion

Various traditional and digital self-tracking methods are available to help individuals take control and reduce health-related anxieties today. However, these methods can influence self-perception, feelings of safety, and social relationships, including family bonds. They can shape health norms, such as the portrayal of an idealised health image on social media. Furthermore, the widespread use and commercialisation of wearable devices and self-help applications may negatively impact perceptions of the body, self, health, and professional support such as psychotherapy. The challenges related to direct access to one's bodily and self-experience, which highlight the limitations and contradictions of the QS approach, are also significant in today's context. Sociopolitical factors, personal biases, and scientific perspectives influence the algorithms that record and interpret measurement outcomes. In self-tracking, well-being, health, and happiness are often reduced to specific ideal values that reflect societal stereotypes, putting pressure on users to alter their behaviour to meet these standards. Such norms do not apply equally to everyone and disproportionately impact marginalised groups, including gender and sexual minorities, ethnic minorities, and indigenous populations. Recognising the complex nature of digital systems is essential, and awareness must be raised so that experiences vary considerably across different societal groups. This underscores the importance of expanding qualitative research into lived experiences, alongside professional guidance and reliable information.

5

UNCERTAINTIES AROUND HEALTHY EATING

Food and eating are significant areas of health anxiety for many individuals. From childhood, we learn that proper nutrition is fundamental to health and safety. Furthermore, food shapes our understanding of reward and punishment, desire and restraint, as well as control and discipline. Our language is rich with metaphors related to eating; for example, we often describe our emotional states using terms like ‘sweet’, ‘bitter’, ‘sugar’, and ‘honey’. In some experiences, we must ‘digest’; in others, we cannot ‘swallow’ (Roberts, 1998). For many individuals, including parents and carers, eating has become a complex challenge that can provoke anxiety. The focus shifts from the sensory and social aspects of eating to concerns about food ingredients, portion sizes, meal schedules, and consumption patterns. These worries about food often reflect more profound existential anxieties regarding identity, body image, social status, ageing, and mortality.

Knowledge and perceptions of food and health involve a variety of individual interpretations, often filled with contradictions, frustrations, and cognitive dissonance which characterise modern social views – not just about nutrition but also about one’s overall social role and healthy behaviour (Chamberlain, 2004; Chrzan & Cargill, 2022). It is well known that food can help reduce anxiety. This spans from the comforting experience of shared meals in infancy to the disturbances in eating behaviours found in bulimia and other eating disorders. Historically, many fasting, dieting, and eating rituals have served to manage and alleviate anxiety, often guided by religious rules and practices. In today’s secular and globalised societies, the consumer industry predominantly takes on this role, including food, health, and pharmaceuticals. Entire subcultures have emerged around fad diets, with specific customs, rules, and designated ‘priests’ such as consultants, therapists, and gurus (Ladyka et al., 2023). The rhetoric surrounding diets that promise quick results for weight loss or other health goals appeals to our desire for easy,

DOI: 10.4324/9781003517788-5

straightforward solutions to the insecurities brought about by an abundance of information, our divergence from social ideals, and concerns about our health and safety (Baldemor et al., 2024; Spadine & Patterson, 2022). A major influence on this discourse is the media, particularly social media, which utilises various tools of 'foodfluencing' (Bayram et al., 2024; Dane & Bhatia, 2023).

In this chapter, I will first analyse the role of the media in science communication and the impact of social stereotypes and prejudices on anxieties related to food and health. I will illustrate this through the intriguing case of a specific symptom complex called 'Chinese restaurant syndrome' (CRS). This narrative serves as a case study to illustrate how diverse social and cultural factors, environmental influences, and shifts in consumer habits impact our relationship with food and occasionally lead to biased attitudes towards the gastronomy of other nations. These factors influence our perceptions of what is healthy, safe, or even dangerous and how they relate to health anxiety, both as a cause and a consequence.

The rise and fall of the 'Chinese restaurant syndrome'

In January 2020, the Japanese company Ajinomoto, a major producer of monosodium glutamate (MSG), launched a global campaign urging the editors of the Merriam-Webster dictionary to redefine the term 'Chinese restaurant syndrome' (Nierenberg, 2020). They proposed that the dictionary replace the original description with a new definition, highlighting that 'Chinese restaurant syndrome' is outdated and unfairly associates Chinese food containing MSG with various physical symptoms. This news was published in *The New York Times*, and its significance extended beyond correcting a scientific or medical error; it aimed to address the xenophobic and, some would argue, racist connotations of the term. This initiative also aimed to mitigate the business interests tied to the marketing of MSG. In response, the editors of Merriam-Webster clarified that they do not create, endorse, or specifically sanction any terms but record the evolution of language (Nierenberg, 2020). Interestingly, 52 years earlier, in 1968, *The New York Times* had also been a significant media player in disseminating the 'Chinese restaurant syndrome' concept and reinforcing corresponding perceptions and attitudes (Lyons, 1968).

On 4 April 1968, a Chinese-American physician, Robert Ho Man Kwok, reported in the *New England Journal of Medicine* that he had experienced numbness, weakness and increased heart palpitations after eating in Chinese restaurants (Kwok, 1968). Letters poured into the journal from reputable physicians describing similar symptoms they had experienced. Two months later, *The New York Times* published an article titled '"Chinese Restaurant Syndrome" Puzzles Doctors' (Lyons, 1968). Two years later, the leading scientific journal, *Nature*, published a report suggesting that a widely used flavour enhancer, MSG, was responsible for the symptoms (Morselli & Grattini, 1970). Nutritionists have largely argued that, in many cases, the symptoms may be due to different combinations of compounds or previously unrecognised food allergies rather than MSG or psychological causes (Metcalfe et al., 2013). Despite reassurances from experts, many people who had experienced symptoms after eating Chinese food remained uneasy. They would have preferred a known cause for these medically unexplained complaints. Although scientific and popular discussions eventually faded, the term 'Chinese restaurant syndrome' has persisted in public awareness. Even today, some Chinese restaurants in Western countries display signs reading 'No MSG'. While this information is neutral, the negative phrasing can evoke health concerns, unfavourable perceptions, and avoidance behaviours (Chen, 2024).

Research has shown that lay representations of 'Chinese restaurant syndrome' included symptoms other than those officially described: headache, thirst, dizziness, stomach cramps, diarrhoea, hot flushes, and heart palpitations. However, when explicitly asked about these symptoms, people did not associate them solely with Chinese restaurants (Kerr et al., 1977, 1979). The researchers discovered that the symptoms and the associated beliefs were more indicative of the individuals experiencing the symptoms than of the food they consumed or their eating habits. Nevertheless, there was a widespread belief that MSG in Chinese cuisine was more harmful than in other foods, such as fast food or preserved items. Over time, there were scientific proposals to rename the CRS, but the original name remained for decades (Zanfirescu et al., 2019). This underscores the need to examine the links between social psychological factors, such as stereotypes, prejudice, and associated anxieties.

As reported in the 2020 article in *The New York Times*, Chinese restaurants proliferated in the United States in 1966, following large numbers of refugees arriving after the Chinese Cultural Revolution, most of whom were impoverished (Nierenberg, 2020). Krishnendu Ray, a professor of nutrition at New York University, stated that people's attitudes towards refugees are closely linked to how they perceive their culture and cuisine (Yam, 2020). In addition to fears, cultural stereotypes, and prejudices about foreigners, a 'buy cheap, pay dear' mentality may also contribute to resentment and ambivalence regarding the reliability and quality of inexpensive restaurants. The fear of exotic, foreign cuisines has existed in countries where immigrants settled and opened restaurants since the late 19th century. Since then, the situation has undergone significant changes, with multicultural gastronomy gaining increasing popularity. Despite numerous changes over the years that have made cuisines from different cultures more appealing, it's surprising that the term 'Chinese restaurant syndrome' has persisted for so long. One possible explanation is that this term has become a catch-all for various concerns and fears associated with unexplained digestive symptoms. This may also explain why some people were not only surprised but also disappointed when it was revealed a few years ago that the entire 'Chinese restaurant syndrome' narrative was based on a scientific hoax and misunderstandings propagated by the media.

In 1968, following the publication of the original Kwok letter, many sceptical responses appeared in the *New England Journal of Medicine* regarding the validity of the so-called 'Chinese restaurant syndrome' (Mosby, 2009). However, a notable shift in perspective emerged only after 2013, when rhetorical scholar Jennifer L. LeMesurier began to analyse the Kwok letter and its responses (LeMesurier, 2017). She discovered that these texts often carried an ironic tone. Her rhetorical analysis revealed that these letters belong to a genre known as 'comic syndrome letters' (CSL), which medical linguists identify as subtly mocking genuine scientific communication and the scientific dilemmas and uncertainties it entails (Hunter, 1990). A vital characteristic of these 'comic syndrome letters' is their striking similarity in style and content to authentic medical 'syndrome letters', as both address uncertain, medically unexplained symptoms and previously unreported drug side effects (Hunter, 2020). The editors of the *New England Journal of Medicine* likely knew that the Kwok letter published in 1968 was a joke. The misconception about CRS originated with an article published in *The New York Times* two months later (Lyons, 1968). Interestingly, this article not only influenced the attitudes and anxieties of the public but also prompted doctors and researchers to seriously investigate and 'prove' the harmful effects of MSG, particularly in the food served in Chinese restaurants. Notably, one of the authors of responses to the joke letter, Herbert Schaumburg, later published a study in *Science* that examined the reality of CRS based on experimental evidence (Schaumburg et al., 1969).

The story's most exciting and revealing twist occurred in 2018 when Jennifer L. LeMesurier received a phone call from Dr Howard Steel. He disclosed that he was behind the name 'Ho Man Kwok' and the CRS hoax in 1968 (Blanding, 2019). During the call, he shared that as a young orthopaedic surgeon with little scientific background, he had made a $10 bet with another doctor, claiming that he could publish an article in a prestigious journal like the *New England Journal of Medicine*. Dr Steel passed away shortly after that conversation at the age of 97. However, his intention to reveal his identity and address the issue of 'Chinese restaurant syndrome' was accomplished.

In 2020, several leading international news outlets reported on the campaign to abolish the term 'Chinese restaurant syndrome', including a story that uncovered Dr Ho Man Kwok's identity (China Daily Global, 2020). This may have contributed to the fact that the Merriam-Webster dictionary now lists CRS as an 'outdated, sometimes offensive' label and suggests the name 'MSG (monosodium glutamate) syndrome' (Merriam-Webster Dictionary, n.d.). In this sense, the story has a happy ending. However, it is not easy to conclude when one considers the individuals who have embraced the biased belief systems shaped mainly by the media and, to some extent, by science, over the past half-century or more. This may have influenced their health anxiety and beliefs related to symptoms, potentially leading to a more negative impact on their attitudes and fears regarding Chinese food and culture. This ripple effect is reflected in the recent public call by a coalition of community activists for the *New England Journal of Medicine* to reconsider its past role in perpetuating negative stereotypes about Chinese food (Chen, 2024).

The gluten-free debate

As the story above illustrates, food is a highly sensitive topic in public communication. This sensitivity is particularly pronounced regarding food intolerances and allergies, which have increased significantly in recent decades and may play a key role in the development and intensification of health anxieties (Lyons & Forde, 2004; Polloni & Muraro, 2020). This topic has garnered considerable public and media attention (Jones, 2020). Gluten sensitivity is a prominent example of the complex bio-psycho-social interrelationships of food intolerances, sensitivities, and associated health anxieties. There are two forms. The first is *coeliac disease*, a chronic, genetically determined immune system disorder that has been recognised by medical science for a long time (Freeman, 2015). The second, known as *non-coeliac syndrome*, is a digestive disorder with similar symptoms of bloating, diarrhoea, and abdominal discomfort, which many people also associate with the consumption of gluten-containing foods. However, coeliac disease and wheat sensitivity are not medically detectable in these cases (Cárdenas-Torres et al., 2021). In recent years, the prevalence of non-coeliac gluten sensitivity has increased significantly. Medical research has produced conflicting conclusions about the causes of this sharp rise in complaints (Roszkowska et al., 2019). In particular, the diagnostic process is complicated by the fact that many people present with a wide range of abdominal symptoms and self-report as gluten-sensitive (Sergi et al., 2021). Nearly all articles agree that further research is essential to clarify the complex underlying mechanisms. However, the rising prevalence of health issues and the associated anxiety highlight the impact of social factors, particularly the media (Dane & Bhatia, 2023). Researchers also emphasise that sociocultural influences have led many people to adopt gluten-free diets despite evidence of gluten intolerance, which may lead to digestive problems due to imbalanced nutrient intake (Norwood, 2021; Sergi et al., 2021).

A few decades ago, gluten sensitivity was not widely discussed, but that has changed significantly in recent years. Global consumption of gluten-free products was valued at $5.72 billion in 2021 and is projected to reach $9.99 billion by 2028 (Fortune Business Insights, 2022). For example, nearly 30% of the population in the United States has tried some form of a gluten-free diet. The percentage is even higher among younger generations (Collins, 2022). Many people are trying to lose weight or 'cure' various diseases by following a gluten-free diet, as evidenced by the fact that 65% of respondents in one survey said that gluten-free foods were healthier than those containing gluten, a trend confirmed by several studies (Jones, 2017; Zerbini et al., 2024). As a recent review study has pointed out, there is considerable diversity in lay perceptions about gluten and significant gaps in lay knowledge regarding gluten-free products and labelling (Hassan et al., 2024). The increase in awareness and rising uncertainty and anxiety may primarily stem from the overwhelming amount of information and various media influences. This includes the repeated announcements by high-profile celebrities declaring their gluten intolerance (Jackson, 2023; Norwood, 2021). Similarly, concerns have been heightened, for example, by an internationally published pop science bestselling book informing the public that gluten consumption can cause a range of diseases and symptoms, including autism, dementia, and Alzheimer's disease (Perlmutter, 2016).

As an example of another dietary practice, the significant influence of the media is also evident in the case of the low-carb Atkins diet. Although this diet has several controversial medical aspects and was introduced in the 1960s, it gained widespread popularity in 2000. This surge in interest can largely be attributed to the increasing rates of obesity and type 2 diabetes, along with public discussions about these health issues (Mahdi, 2006). Some of this has also contributed to the gluten-free trend, as many people mistakenly identify gluten, a protein, as a carbohydrate (Chrzan & Cargill, 2022). In international examples, in Italy, for example, two million families buy gluten-free products, but only 170,000 have a family member with a coeliac condition (Sale&Pepe, n.d.). In Hungary and Romania, 22% of households had purchased gluten-free products in the year before the survey, although only 2.5% reported a family member with gluten sensitivity (Szűcs et al., 2019), In other words, nine out of10 households bought gluten-free foods despite there being no evidence of gluten causing any harm. It's worth noting that in the United States, sales of gluten-free products doubled between 2011 and 2014 (Mansharamani, 2015). This increase seems to be primarily influenced by advertising and the media, particularly the rise of social media platforms like Instagram, which gained popularity starting in 2010. Surveys have indicated that the primary motivations include weight loss, healthier living, and avoiding unspecified harmful ingredients (Stephens, 2014). Nevertheless, while digestive disorders or other symptoms associated with gluten were not necessarily the primary reason for adopting this diet, many discovered that a wide range of symptoms were alleviated or eliminated by following a gluten-free regimen (Niland & Cash, 2018). In addition, many people have reported that when they returned to eating gluten-containing foods, their symptoms returned, either in their original form or in a modified form. These reactions can be partly explained by the established psychological fact that expectations significantly influence symptom formation; we are more likely to notice symptoms when we anticipate them. Research indicates that even the name given to an illness can affect how individuals perceive their symptoms and impact their experience (Petrie & Weinman, 2017). Researchers have attributed this phenomenon to the *nocebo effect*, in which the expectation of harm – such as experiencing unpleasant sensations, symptoms, or even illness – can lead to increased anxiety and heightened awareness of negative bodily sensations (Rooney et al., 2023). This, in turn, may contribute to the formation of symptoms, along with the social context – including gender, class, and the availability of alternatives. The quality and source of information are crucial in the development of the *nocebo effect* and are closely linked to health anxiety (Grosso et al., 2024).

Undoubtedly, gluten intolerance is a genuine issue and can lead to significant distress for those affected. The reality that only the coeliac form has been empirically substantiated does not imply that the non-coeliac form cannot have a medical basis nor that the individuals involved are not experiencing suffering. Unfortunately, numerous non-coeliac patients are labelled as having 'imaginary' or 'psychological' symptoms. Professionals and laypeople must recognise that stress, health beliefs, fears, and expectations can contribute to symptoms. Even if the biomedical paradigm has not proven what causes symptoms in non-coeliac gluten-sensitive individuals, we must accept that these symptoms exist, that people suffer, and that they deserve assistance (Lebwohl & Leffler, 2015). To do this, however, it is crucial to understand that the social influences affecting individual beliefs, fears, and behaviours are embedded in complex cultural and religious belief systems that date back thousands of years. These can have a significant, if unconscious, impact on dietary habits. An understanding of this socio-cultural-historical background can also contribute significantly to a better understanding of the underlying causes and psychological demands of medically unexplained gluten sensitivity and other food intolerances and to reducing the associated health anxiety.

'Harmful' civilisation, 'dangerous' food?

Though gluten intolerance seems relatively recent, even ancient Taoist 'grain-free' monks in China claimed that their diet could cure diseases (Chrzan & Cargill, 2022). It is an interesting paradox that grains were symbols of the sophistication of contemporary Chinese civilisation and agricultural culture. However, it was precisely against the evils of modernisation that the early Taoists took a stand, recognising early on the potential drawbacks of civilisation alongside its developmental benefits (Levinovitz, 2015). In public discourse within contemporary societies, various actors in the food industry frequently emphasise that their products are free from the dangers of modern civilisation and artificial substances that can be harmful to health. Rhetorically, they support this by saying that their food is 'natural' or by scapegoating a 'dangerous' ingredient. They often propagate that their product does not contain that ingredient and is therefore 'safe', that is 'pure', 'organic', 'non-processed', and 'clean'. However, a common consequence of this is that 'clean' diets, if not carefully chosen, are not supported by medical and dietary studies, and only promoted by the media and social media, can lead to digestive problems and even eating disorders (Ambwani et al., 2019). Individuals concerned about potential adverse effects may have an unbalanced diet or restrict their food intake. Clinical observations also confirm that a significant proportion of patients with eating disorders start with some form of food taboo or avoidant behaviour (Wróblewska et al., 2018).

In public discussions about food, both artificial ingredients and various natural nutrients – such as salt, fat, carbohydrates, sugar, gluten, and lactose – have been identified as sources of danger and anxiety. Many people filter out the 'dangerous substances' that cause them anxiety and remove them from their diets based on the media or social communication. Anxiety often manifests as physical symptoms, especially digestive issues, creating a cycle where nearly any food may increase anxiety and lead to further problems. This can lead people to extreme diets, some of which are harmful to their health. A notable example is singer Madonna's 'air diet', discussed in Grazia, which involves consuming 'water soup' to mimic eating (The Frisky, 2010). Such extreme rituals can be seen psychologically, not merely as responses to celebrity trends but as methods for individuals to gain control. By avoiding 'dangerous' foods, they can alleviate anxiety. Moreover, these rituals connect people to behavioural trends, reinforcing the perceived value of specific practices. This need for control may stem from a desire to alleviate anxiety through tangible experiences.

Research suggests that many individuals perceive the consumption of convenience foods, canned goods, and fast food as excessive and 'untrustworthy'. As a substitute, they often turn to a gluten-free or other 'clean' diet, which they mistakenly consider 'natural' (Gibson et al., 2017). There are many different views, beliefs, and anxieties about naturalness. These often reflect a desire to address anxieties about modernity, the influence of technological civilisation, and the contradictions in scientific information (Bauman, 2006). The soothing effect of consuming 'safe' foods links to research showing that lactose-free milk drinkers often feel calm and positive (Castellini & Graffigna, 2022). This stems from the belief that milk is safe and healthy. While lactose intolerance affects more people than gluten intolerance, many who drink lactose-free milk are not intolerant. Surveys indicate that these consumers typically have higher income and education levels, demonstrating confidence in food science and knowledge of healthy, 'safe' diets and lifestyles (Gulseven & Wohlgenant, 2017). People with various food allergies and/or who eat 'clean' tend to have these characteristics. This also highlights that sociocultural and psychological influences are significant factors in developing these behaviours, alongside the effects of manufacturers and retailers. These factors also affect how consumers perceive labels and pictograms on 'clean' foods (Amos et al., 2014). Many individuals view these labels as symbols of naturalness, providing a positive emotional affirmation that the product is safe and healthy. This belief persists even when the label is fictitious, as demonstrated in a study by Priven et al. (2015) on the construction of 'MUI-free' products, a name coined by the researchers.

Many take pride in affording 'clean' products, reinforcing their health-conscious identity. 'Free from' labels appear on food packaging and in bakeries, cafes, and restaurants, promoting products and suggesting that the establishment is 'healthy and safe'. The reassurance from food labels partly arises from fear of unrecognisable ingredients. For example, gluten, found in everyday foods like bread and beer, is also present in thickeners such as those used in soups and serves as a moisture barrier in spices and stamp glue. This can make gluten seem like a hidden danger everywhere. Such fear extends to social interactions, including worrying about offending others with food offers, how to decline lunch invitations, and whether suitable 'safe' food options are available when travelling. It raises the challenge of prioritising personal interests over others': are friendship and social life more important than feeling safe?

Swedish ethnologist Kristofer Hansson calls the spaces our bodies perceive as unsafe 'critical spaces' (Hansson, 2020). In these spaces, tension arises from the conflict between the social benefits that the space offers (e.g. the pleasure of meeting friends) and the perceived danger (being offered food that we do not want to eat). Many people, therefore, seek out safe spaces and 'safe' companies where people share similar eating habits and are not exposed to the dangers of food or its socio-communicative anxieties (Thomas & Cankurt, 2024).

Nourishing bonds: food, safety, and identity

Eating habits, diets, and rituals provide security and opportunities for shared thoughts and discussions (Dunbar, 2017). They help develop both personal and group identities and establish boundaries, which can reduce anxiety (Fox & Ward, 2008). American religious scholar Benjamin Zeller describes strict 'clean' and 'pure' eating habits, along with the communities that form around them, as practices that build a sense of community and function similar to religion (Zeller, 2015). He argues that individuals seek new ways to form communal identities in the consumer-driven Western world of late modernity, where traditional religious practices have diminished. This allows them to connect and find transcendent meanings, thereby gaining social support and a sense of purpose and safety in an increasingly complex and anxious world. According to Zeller (2015), veganism and gluten-free, palaeolithic, raw food, and organic diets give food and eating a transcendent quality. This means that adherents are encouraged to develop a worldview with personal meaning, and rituals and other shared practices are created, allowing community to be built around the practice, which in turn facilitates identity formation and connection to the group.

From a symbolically based cultural anthropological perspective, food can acquire totemic and taboo qualities in various rituals (Douglas, 1966). Sigmund Freud (1913/1989) discussed this concept in *Totem and Taboo*, where he explained that in traditional societies, the totem symbolises the tribe: it can be an object or an animal that commands respect and a certain degree of fear. Freud argued that tribes do not destroy the totem; instead, they treat it as a taboo, endowing it with sacred, holy, ghostly, and dangerous meanings, as well as notions of the forbidden and the impure. For the community, the taboo is primarily expressed through prohibitions and restrictions, which serve to foster a sense of belonging and reduce anxiety unconsciously. A special diet may also fulfil this function by providing a tabooed 'totem food' that unites the community and fosters a sense of safety. This communal, supportive function may be the unconscious reason why, for example, a popular restaurant in New York has a name that refers to the taboo *Taboonette*. Many online instances link 'taboo' with eating, suggesting that abstaining from a taboo ingredient becomes a totem. Entire subcultures often form around this, promising wholeness, health, and happiness. Adherents see the diet as vital for health and well-being, linking it with virtues. Control and identity are central to their relationship with 'totem' foods. Zeller (2015) notes that in Western culture, taboo foods include gluten for gluten-free dieters, meat for vegans, and certain 'civilisational foods' for Palaeolithic dieters. This classification is narrow; only those actively involved in these diet movements are categorised through behaviours like attending related events or being part of communities shaping their dietary identity.

This system of tabooed habits may relate to food, the desire to belong to a community, and disillusionment with traditional institutions. Parallels can be drawn, for instance, with individuals who feel disillusioned by conventional healthcare due to inadequate care, impersonality, poor communication, and various other issues; they often turn to alternative healers instead of confronting the 'coldness' associated with academic institutions (Guillaud et al., 2020). Equally, the anxiety-inducing effect of the lack of transparency of the vast amount of expert information on diets may be causing many to flee to alternative diets and seek out safe, protective groups. The motive to seek safety and alleviate anxiety may also be linked to the fact that when someone is unable to achieve the 'perfect' diet, they often punish themselves with various restrictions such as consuming only detox tea, inducing vomiting, or depriving themselves of pleasurable activities like watching films or socialising with friends. These are maladaptive ways of reducing anxiety, and, in many cases, they can become a persistent and further symptomatic tool.

Belonging to a diet group can be a fragile yet intense pillar of personal identity (Babic et al., 2014). This is supported, for example, by the common themes of community, identity, salvation, and spirituality in social media, promoting different diets. Pasi Falk (1994), in his book *The Consuming Body*, relates the notion of an eating community to the bodily connection between consumption, self-construction, and identity formation, attributing to this the strong identity-forming and community-cohesive power of eating. The reciprocity of bodies, along with the solidarity, community, and sharing that can be fostered in this way, also has a potent anti-anxiety effect. Others emphasise the importance of lifestyle and, thus, the separation of social groups, citing the Palaeolithic diet as an example, which is not only a rather expensive dietary trend but also a controlled lifestyle for a higher social class. In the Palaeolithic and many other dietary trends, there is a nature-centredness, a desire to return to origins, a reference to 'paradise', and a state of freedom from anxiety, sometimes with a rather masculine tone: 'Live as the caveman lived' (Williams, 2014).

As we have seen above, diets based on food intolerance are partly community-building, creating groups and self-help communities and thus having an anti-anxiety function. Nevertheless, they also individualise dining experiences and create social boundaries, as individuals outside the group cannot partake in the same food. This can also be the source of the ongoing, but not necessarily conscious, tension behind different eating practices, and it is this tension that serves to create a dependency on dieting, as both eating and deprivation rituals have an anti-anxiety effect.

From orthorexia to anxiety-free eating habits

Concerns about healthy eating are widespread, amplified by media and internet coverage, leading to medicalisation. Over two decades, orthorexia nervosa – considered a severe form of concern about healthy eating – has been identified, though not classified as a disease (Horovitz & Argyrides, 2023). It involves an obsession with healthy foods, which, despite the benefits of healthy eating, can cause physical and mental health problems when excessive. People with orthorexia fixate on food quality and purity, resulting in restrictive habits and social withdrawal. Orthorexia means 'eating right' and was first described by Steven Bratman (Bratman, 1997). The term 'nervosa' clearly refers to its anxiety-related nature. Bratman initially thought that it was only his clientele of alternative medicine practitioners who suffered from the disorder. Still, it turns out that many people are almost obsessive about what, when, where, and how much they eat and that this eventually reaches such proportions that it endangers their well-being. For example, they spend hours a day on their diets, eliminate entire food groups from their diets, develop anxiety about many foods, and develop body image issues. Bratman described the process as beginning with a motivation to eliminate a disease or maintain good health. However, because it is not easy to stick to a diet, the frustration often leads to arrogance towards those who eat 'without discipline'. According to Bratman (1997), the self-justification required to endure hardship in adhering to a strict diet reinforces an individual's belief that they are justified in being cautious about what they eat. And the need for further validation creates the assumption that this is the only truth and the right thing to do.

Estimating the number of people affected by orthorexia can be challenging. However, some experts believe that there may be more cases of orthorexia than of anorexia and bulimia combined. Additionally, various multi-country surveys indicate that the prevalence of orthorexia is steadily increasing, with estimates suggesting that it could be as high as 27% (López et al., 2023; van Dyke, 2018). It is difficult to define when to call this problem a disorder, given the almost endemic guilt in Western culture about eating the 'wrong' foods. This is partly due to the increasing variety of foods available, growing awareness of environmental pollution, and the marketing of 'toxins' and 'superfoods'. The food industry also employs this tactic to produce unhealthy foods, thereby encouraging ongoing consumption. Western societies are heavily exposed to junk food advertising and have easy access to online takeaway services. Nonetheless, individuals are often blamed for choosing to eat them.

Health anxiety and beliefs about the controllability of health have also been shown to be predictors of orthorexia (Greville-Harris et al., 2022). We speak of orthorexia when feelings of guilt and anxiety escalate to the point where the issue of dietary cleanliness slowly becomes more important than any other value, affecting everyday behaviour, including work and social relationships. As discussed above, anxiety may also be underpinned by an unconscious symbolic representation that food is not only a source of energy but also a protector of the integrity of the body and that eating 'unclean' or 'dangerous' food may threaten the boundaries of the body and the self and even the wider community (Douglas, 1966; Walsh & Baker, 2020). In this sense, eating 'clean' (safe, pure, natural) also becomes a moral imperative, and this is partly where the guilt and intense anxiety that underlie orthorexia come from. It also explains why social and cultural factors so strongly influence this behaviour.

Contrary to popular belief, orthorexia is not just a problem for young girls but also can affect anyone (Strahler, 2019). However, it can manifest differently in women and men, with orthorexia being equally prevalent in both sexes but not always visible to the public and men's problems being less socially visible and acceptable. According to philosopher and cultural studies scholar Susan Bordo, every era since the dawn of modernity has exhibited an emblematic behavioural disorder that illustrates how social pressures to constrain women, particularly, are 'written on bodies' (Bordo, 2004). While women were labelled hysterical in the early 20th century, agoraphobia became 'fashionable' in the 1950s, especially in the United States, where middle-class women were expected to stay at home instead. Then, in the 1980s, anorexia became more prevalent, expressing a desire for women to look less conspicuous in the corporate world. Following this line of thought, in recent years, 'clean eating' can be seen as being used to curb cravings and ward off and mask anxiety. This may also stem from stereotypical expectations that health for men is associated with notions of strength and endurance. In contrast, it is related to notions of attractiveness and energy for women. For women, appetite must be 'controlled', always 'watching the lines'. The 'hungry woman' is also 'unseemly' and 'dangerous' in other ways, whereas for men, this is not the case; a man can be ravenous, and this even reinforces the image of masculinity. According to traditional gender stereotypes, men need to 'build up' their bodies to be bigger, stronger, and faster. This is why a man may prefer to eat meat, while a vegetarian man sometimes needs to prove his masculinity. Although traditional cultural beliefs and social expectations concerning men and women have evolved significantly in recent years, gender stereotypes continue to persist. This is evident when you search for the term 'orthorexia' in Google Image Search, as most images that appear feature women.

Several social scientists contend that the focus on food and diet arises from recognising that these domains represent significant areas of autonomy, identity, and control in contemporary globalised consumer societies, offering opportunities for individual choice and separation from others (Ilanganu-Bresch, 2020). Orthorexia is also a socially accepted behaviour, as it implies healthy behaviour and 'pure' eating, for which no one can be criticised or questioned. The clean eating trend aligns with the digital revolution, which has led to many websites, apps, blogs, and social media platforms providing advice on maintaining a healthy lifestyle. Of all the digital platforms, Instagram is the one that is having the most significant impact on orthorexia behaviour. In one study, it was found that 49% of Instagram users scored highly on the orthorexia scale (Turner & Lefevre, 2017). There is an uncontrollable and unstoppable influx of photos of 'healthy' food, images of 'perfect' bodies on social media, and various advertisements. In this sense, orthorexia also becomes a kind of public performance, promoting purity and naturalness under the banner of health consciousness, as opposed to what mass culture considers to be artificial, toxic, junk products (Hanganu-Bresch, 2020). The question, of course, is how natural the products advertised as organic are. This elusive question is confusing for many, so fears and reactions to food are widespread.

The cornerstones of the public discourse on healthy eating are often set along forced oppositions: natural/synthetic, organic/genetically modified, whole grain/refined, and genuine/artificial. As we have seen above, these are accompanied by moral content, and ethical imperatives demand a commitment to a 'pure' state, that is a perfectly healthy diet. The anxiety is heightened by the fact that the boundaries of what is deemed healthy are not clearly defined and can be extended indefinitely. There is also the question of whether the global problems of 'uncleanliness' (mass consumption, pollution, climate crisis) and the associated anxiety can be addressed by individual solutions to the quest for safety. However, on an individual level, practising mindful eating can help develop a balanced relationship with food and reduce anxiety by focusing on the pleasurable aspects of eating rather than the ingredients themselves (Christodoulou et al., 2024a). It counters social media's negative body ideals by promoting empowerment and a relaxation of rigid views. Although challenging due to complex factors, evidence-based techniques can strengthen trust between communities and professionals. This enables individuals to access expert advice; connect with supportive groups; and develop healthy, enjoyable eating habits. Building trust in science and professionals, as well as sharing best practices, can promote balance and reduce anxiety.

Conclusion

This chapter explored how our cultural context influences eating habits, and how these habits, in turn, can shape health anxiety as a way of seeking safety. Many individuals remove 'dangerous substances' that provoke anxiety from their diets, often due to stereotypes, biases, or mixed messages from the media and social groups. Food choices are connected to psychological needs through shared stories about safety, identity, and social status associated with being 'fit and healthy'. This is driven by a desire to return to an idealised sense of 'naturalness' amidst the challenges of global industrialisation, as well as the pursuit of spiritual purification. Various factors influence dietary habits, including exposure to social and traditional media, aggressive marketing by producers and retailers targeting consumers, and advice from medical literature and mainstream sources that highlight certain health benefits. People may exclude specific ingredients for reasons such as alleviating gastrointestinal symptoms or other health issues or due to the belief that these ingredients are harmful, making dietary restrictions seem healthier.

Furthermore, in many Western societies, individuals are often blamed for choosing to eat 'unhealthy' foods, even though these are made easily available by the food industry. A thorough analysis is needed to explore ways to reduce the food industry's influence on our food choices, examine the links between gender and power dynamics, and emphasise the importance of trusting evidence-based professional guidance to foster balanced, anxiety-free relationships with food.

6

RESPONSIBILITY AND BLAME IN HEALTH AND ILLNESS

It is well known that illness, loss of health, and feelings of weakness and vulnerability can significantly increase fear and anxiety. Less well known, however, is the sense of responsibility and, in many cases, guilt and self-blame associated with the onset of illness, which can have a similar effect. In today's societies, the pressure on the individual to maintain control, efficiency, and responsibility is often overemphasised. This societal expectation, embodied in slogans such as 'It's all in the mind' or 'You just have to want it, and you'll get better', can often become a catalyst for further health anxiety and significantly impair both health behaviour and recovery.

Stress, illness, and self-blame: vicious circles?

The concept of victim-blaming, related to 'healthism', has been a topic within health psychology and sociology since the 1970s (Crawford, 1977, 1980). However, it is only in recent decades that the issue of self-blame, partly stemming from victim-blaming, has been systematically explored. Some have examined it within the context of social psychological attributions and implicit theories, which relate individual behaviour and decisions to blame and social support (Dohle et al., 2022). Others have done so within the context of self-criticism, guilt, shame, and stigma, which are linked to the strong emphasis in Western societies on concepts of risk, population health, and individual lifestyle (Akbari et al., 2023; Callebaut et al., 2016; Martin, 2001). Research tends to start from the premise that when any unexpected adverse life event occurs, most people seek explanations for what might have caused it and what factors may have contributed to the problem. It is not uncommon to look for the fault, the 'culprit', in oneself. Often, an illness presents a situation we have not encountered before, forcing us to make decisions we

DOI: 10.4324/9781003517788-6

have never faced before. Many individuals find it challenging to decide and recover because they cannot escape the anxiety-provoking question: what is the reason, and who is responsible for putting me in this situation?

Most individuals face questions of this nature, either directly or through family members, as life expectancy rises, and many reach the age at which they are most likely to develop an illness. According to international statistics, chronic diseases are the leading cause of death, accounting for nearly 68% of deaths according to some estimates (Hacker, 2024; Jannati et al., 2020). However, it is not always easy to determine which factors in health behaviour may contribute to a disease, and to what extent responsibility rests with the individual. Other factors such as, for example, quality of life have also been identified as being particularly significant influences on the self-blame of chronic patients, such as those with chronic obstructive pulmonary disease (COPD), which affects 15 to 20% of smokers (Woo et al., 2021).

Responsibility involves recognising and following the proper behaviour to stay healthy or recover. Taking the blame for developing a disease can lead to self-blame, causing distress and health anxiety. While it is commonly believed that self-blame increases stress, this is not always true (Callebaut et al., 2016). Blaming one's past behaviours and linking them to the illness tend to have less negative impact compared to what is known as *characterological self-blame* (Taebi et al., 2021). In the latter case, individuals may attribute their illness to their personality traits. For example, someone might blame themselves for being lazy and therefore unable to lose weight, ultimately attributing their heart attack to this perceived lack of effort. Similarly, it is common for one partner in a couple to take on the blame for unsuccessful pregnancies, with women tending to do so more frequently (Péloquin et al., 2017). This self-blame can lead to a devaluation of their own personality and character, as well as a diminished sense of femininity (Taebi et al., 2021). This type of self-blame is more intense because we often perceive our character as stable while viewing our behaviour as changeable. Other authors argue that individuals with a higher quality of life tend to be less inclined to blame themselves for developing diseases (Cho et al., 2022). Conversely, self-blame can also influence the quality of life. For instance, a follow-up study found that cardiology patients with higher levels of characterological self-blame exhibited a higher rate of disease symptom deterioration, thus negatively impacting their quality of life (Harry et al., 2015).

Studies indicate that patients who attribute setbacks to a lack of ability or weaknesses in their skills display heightened stress responses in various illnesses (Dweck, 2000; Jannati et al., 2020). Additionally, stronger stress responses were noted in instances where self-blame was connected to behavioural and character traits as well (Plaufcan et al., 2012). Similarly, it should be considered that self-blame can be as much a consequence as a cause of illness-related stress and anxiety. In several studies, particularly in cancer patients, it has been found that the stress of the disease itself was a trigger for self-blame (Bennett et al., 2005; Jannati et al., 2020). However, it is more likely that these two factors interact. When individuals blame themselves, they become self-critical and develop a negative self-image, worsening their mood and impairing health management, relationships, family functioning, and quality of life. Reinforcing self-compassion – encompassing empathy, compassion, and self-acceptance – can reduce self-criticism and self-blame (Golden, 2024; Meerholz et al., 2019). This can be a significant challenge in contemporary societies where social media perpetuates an idealised notion of perfection and happiness. However, if the client can accept that being human also encompasses vulnerability and imperfections, they will be less inclined to blame themselves for their shortcomings such as illness. This, in turn, can reduce anxiety, which also contributes to maintaining better health.

Self-blame and associated anxiety are also interconnected with body image and self-image. Clinical experience and research indicate that patients often experience feelings of shame and conceal their bodies, viewing themselves as less valuable and acceptable to the outside world (Duncan & Cacciatore, 2015). In extreme cases, self-deprecation and self-blame may be accompanied by a withdrawal from coping with the illness, leading to frustration, apathy, and a state of learnt helplessness (Seligman, 1975). This frequently occurs alongside intense anxiety, anger, and hostility towards the environment, usually the treatment staff. The patient may feel that 'no one understands my situation' or that 'everyone minds their own business'. This can lead to conflicts with those around them, which may increase feelings of frustration, misunderstanding, anxiety, depression, and loneliness. Negative attitudes and self-blame can act as triggers for depression, and the relationship is also reciprocal: individuals who have experienced depression previously tend to react more strongly to the illness with self-blame (Brzozowski & Crossey, 2024). This can also be explained by the 'scar' model of depression, which suggests that new stress can activate the previous depressive response pattern, the previous 'scar' (Steiger et al., 2015). This has been confirmed by brain imaging, specifically fMRI scans: electrical activity in various areas of the brain was observed when guilt was experienced by individuals who had previously suffered from depression, but was not observed in healthy controls (Lythe et al., 2015).

Self-blame has been investigated in a variety of patient populations, with most studies conducted in cancer patients. In these patients, self-reported self-blame for their disease was found to be between 18% and 39% (Pham et al., 2021). However, there were studies in which the prevalence of self-blame in advanced cancer patients was over 50%. On average, 24% of patients with lung cancer experienced strong self-blame. In a study by Milbury et al. (2012), 47% of patients reported strong self-blame, which frequently led to them concealing their disease from those around them. This phenomenon is not isolated from the social stigma that persists about cancer and the identification of cancer as a deadly disease (Castillo & Santa-Cruz-Espinoza, 2024; Huang et al., 2021).

The development of guilt, shame, and self-blame displays a distinctive and dynamic pattern throughout the history of a disease. Research among patients with

COPD has revealed intriguing correlations regarding how patients' self-esteem changed after diagnosis (Halding et al., 2011; Woo et al., 2021). Many patients perceived themselves to be outside the realm of the healthy and did not receive the support they had previously. They often felt discredited because they believed that society had judged their illness to be self-inflicted because they smoked. As a result, patients suffered from negative emotions and tended to hide. The attitudes observed in healthcare settings frequently led to feelings of self-blame and guilt (Berger et al., 2011). Patients reported that their concerns were minimised compared to the topic of smoking even during consultations, where they experienced an otherwise supportive atmosphere. Unsupportive encounters can make it more difficult for patients to cope with the feelings of self-blame and guilt. When patients try to hide their illness by using passive coping strategies, it can further limit their access to peer support, increase the likelihood of critical incidents, and delay necessary medical treatment. Additionally, avoiding help can put smokers with COPD at greater risk. This may contribute significantly to their continued smoking. Feelings of self-blame and exclusion can lead to increased anxiety, which they may try to alleviate by smoking.

Responsibility and victim-blaming

Blaming oneself necessitates a sense of responsibility for the situation and an awareness of the consequences. For instance, in a study conducted in the 1990s, 38% of melanoma patients did not attribute blame to themselves for developing the disease, despite having deliberately sunbathed, indicating that they had not been exposed to the sun 'by accident' (Dirksen, 1995). It became clear that they were unaware of the repercussions of sun exposure. Awareness is significantly greater today, 30 years after the study. However, numerous other factors can influence our perception of fault, including our sense of control over events, our understanding of risk factors, and our belief in the presence of order and justice in the world (Lerner, 1970, 1980). Another key factor is the sense of responsibility we feel for our health and whether we believe that others hold us accountable for our illnesses. In a classic study examining attitudes towards 66 different illnesses and health conditions, researchers found that the degree of personal responsibility attributed to illness predicted participants' social distancing and rejection behaviours (Crandall & Moriarty, 1995). As for specific illnesses, research has indicated that patients with HIV/AIDS and lung cancer often receive less support from those around them, as well as from healthcare professionals, compared to patients with other conditions (Mantler et al., 2003; Schweitzer et al., 2023). This lack of support may stem from societal prejudices and blaming HIV/AIDS patients for their homosexuality and lung cancer patients for smoking. Resentment and anger were more frequently reported by those blamed for their condition than by those only assumed to be responsible but not held accountable. Feeling blamed can deepen self-blame, anxiety, and depression.

Several studies have also investigated the indirect negative impact of attributions, namely blaming, on coping with chronic illness. These studies have found that avoidant coping strategies are most likely to play a role (Gonzalez et al., 2015; Livneh, 2019; Roesch & Weiner, 2001). Avoidant coping reduces anxiety and promotes safety by avoiding problems. Self-blame increases dependence on avoidant strategies, which leads to poor adjustment and hampers safety. Evidence demonstrates that it delays problem-solving and decreases treatment adherence. Conversely, beliefs about health responsibility might reduce avoidant coping and enhance adjustment. This finding aligns with prior research, which shows that self-blame and responsibility have different effects on psychological adjustment (Voth & Sirois, 2009). The differences between self-blame and responsibility were similar to the characterological and behavioural self-blame constructs presented above. Patients who attributed the source of their health condition to themselves rather than to their behaviour were more likely to use avoidant coping strategies, less likely to accept the limitations and difficulties of living with a chronic illness, and less likely to manage illness-related stress effectively (Pham et al., 2021).

The issue of responsibility has three constituent parts: a responsible agent, having obligations, and being liable to be held responsible (Snelling, 2015). In the context of health, all three factors can be problematic and may be associated with health anxiety. The issue of blame also raises the question of the purpose of accountability. For instance, as will be discussed in the subsequent chapter, if obesity is socially unacceptable, it may have a positive health purpose, but this may also lead to blaming people who are overweight (Monaghan et al., 2022). The issue of personal moral responsibility for health is also problematic, even though health-damaging behaviours are generally evidence based (Khan et al., 2021). For instance, it is a well-established fact that a correlation exists between smoking and the incidence of heart attacks. However, it is crucial to acknowledge that not all smokers will necessarily experience heart attacks, and, conversely, non-smokers may still be at risk of this condition. Statistics describe associations by the law of large numbers. However, this only indicates probability and risk in individual cases, not certainty, and other causes also contribute to the disease aside from risk behaviour. Therefore, we cannot definitively claim that smokers are entirely to blame or solely responsible for their condition. Likewise, it cannot be described as a function of preventive risk behaviour who will blame themselves after or even before the onset of the disease. We have seen examples of this during the coronavirus pandemic. A considerable number of personal accounts and articles have been published that describe how many people did not undergo testing or consulted a doctor at an advanced stage of their illness due to the feelings of anxiety that if they were diagnosed, those around them would perceive them as irresponsible and guilty for not taking sufficient precautions (Min, 2021).

While individuals are responsible for their health choices, they cannot be blamed for diseases due to their complex causes, influenced by many factors, including the environment. Personal agency is always situated within a social context, raising questions about dyadic responsibility – how the environment encourages risk behaviours – and diachronic responsibility, which considers responsibility over time (Brown & Savulescu, 2019). This discussion broadens the understanding of responsible health behaviours that also support anxiety-free coping. One crucial element in health promotion and healing is the need for individuals to connect with their future selves. People can make better health choices if they consider how their actions will affect their future well-being and act in ways that benefit their future self (Creutzfeldt & Holloway, 2020). However, many life circumstances and social factors influence the extent to which someone can consider future perspectives. It is also common for someone to struggle with changing a health-damaging behaviour or effectively engaging with health professionals when they become unwell, especially if they lack a clear vision of themselves in the future as healthy or improved. When this positive image is missing or associated with health anxiety, it becomes difficult for the individual to take responsibility for their actions and behaviours.

It is also common to blame patients if they are overly optimistic about their condition. In clinical practice, we frequently encounter the phenomenon of professionals or family members believing that patients do not want to face reality, particularly in the case of end-stage cancer patients (Thomas, 2012). However, they are also blamed for expressing negative feelings and anxieties, which the environment perceives as 'overreacting' to their condition. Another source of blame lies in the belief in the omnipotence of science and professionals (Lakin & Kane, 2022). This belief primarily arises from the frustration and disappointment, often accompanied by anxiety, experienced by the professional, the patient, or the family member, who feels that, despite the enormous potential of advanced medicine today, it cannot cure all diseases (Bell et al., 2002). Frustration is frequently directed towards the patient, who is perceived as the 'weakest link' and is thus held accountable for their behaviour or personal characteristics. This is partly due to a lack of language to accurately distinguish between the complex effects and relationships that influence health. Consequently, professionals and patients often employ the 'intentional/unintentional' dichotomy to describe the context of a problem and the degree to which a person's behaviour contributes to the health issue (Hart et al., 2007). This can even result in victim-blaming, as demonstrated in the case example below.

A few years ago, the public learnt about Resignation Syndrome, also called Traumatic Withdrawal or Abandonment Syndrome, through news reports and the documentary *Life Overtakes Me* (Sallin et al., 2016; Samuelson & Haptas, 2019; Thomas, 2017). Mostly observed in Sweden among Uyghur refugee children and in Nauru, it affects children awaiting immigration status, often amid feelings of hopelessness. The syndrome develops rapidly, characterised by apathy and immobility with no biological explanation (Petrovic, 2016). Many children become catatonic or enter a coma-like state for months or years, requiring care to prevent muscle atrophy. Professionals frequently misunderstand the syndrome and blame parents, particularly mothers, assuming that children learn extreme behaviours from them.

Some scholars argue that hope, mediated by parents, influences recovery (Sallin et al., 2023). Experts view the syndrome differently: some see it as related to apathy, rebellion, or biological factors, while others point out a lack of comprehensive explanations (Kirmayer & Gómez-Camillo, 2019; Makris et al., 2021). Responsibility also plays a part, as feelings of helplessness are central to the syndrome. It also highlights that diagnoses made without a clear understanding often serve as political tools and blame victims at various levels.

Using the 'intentional/unintentional' dimension assists in classifying symptoms without organic causes as 'self-inflicted'. Many patients with unexplained symptoms feel that their condition is not properly recognised (Cheston, 2022), leading to beliefs that they are not receiving adequate care, despite their suffering and frustration (Sallay et al., 2022). Professionals often attribute these symptoms to psychological causes, suggesting traits, behaviour, or poor stress management being the underlying issues, thereby placing full responsibility on patients. These individuals also struggle to articulate their suffering due to a lack of vocabulary and narrative skills, which hampers their ability to present their problems and validate their experiences (Stone, 2014). They often feel ignored or falsely accused of fabricating their complaints. In Western culture, symptoms viewed as 'imagined' are regarded as moral failings (Greco, 1993, 1998), associated with personal choice and responsibility, contrasting with how other patient complaints are perceived (Bensing & Verhaak, 2006).

In contemporary discourses, health risk behaviours are often viewed as the result of an individual's personal history rather than being considered within the broader social and cultural context of their life experiences. While personal experiences are significant, they are not entirely under an individual's control. Factors such as access to healthy food, clean drinking water, adequate rest, exercise, and knowledge about health and illness also play critical roles. Unfortunately, the individualistic approach in psychological and medical practices overshadows these contextual factors. This perspective can create a misleading sense of control and responsibility, resulting in feelings of blame and self-blame.

Post-traumatic growth: challenges and controversies

The relationship between anxiety related to illness, self-blame, and perceptions of safety is multidirectional. To feel secure in the world, it is necessary to maintain a positive attitude that enables us to trust our environment. This attitude has been examined from various psychological perspectives. Classical developmental psychology explains the concept of basic trust, as described by Erikson (1956), while social psychology refers to it as a basic assumption, as discussed by Janoff-Bulman (1992). The basic assumptions theory posits that all our other attitudes and beliefs stem from three core assumptions: the world is benevolent, the world is meaningful, and the self is worthy. However, the world is filled with various external dangers, making the inherent optimism found in basic assumptions and basic trust crucial for individuals to navigate their daily lives with relatively low anxiety levels. The hypothesis of a belief in a just world serves a similar function (Lerner, 1980). Individuals are confronted with adverse events, tragedies, and injustices on a daily basis. To minimise their anxiety regarding these, they utilise compensatory thinking strategies that also focus on safety seeking. Such attributions often result in people blaming the sufferer or victim, which helps them restore a sense of justice in the world and defend against the anxiety of unpredictable and uncontrollable forces. Unfortunately, professionals sometimes adopt the same simplistic explanatory approach without considering its potential impact on the patient or those who have already recovered (Cox & Fritz, 2022). Both the belief in a just world and the basic assumption theory posit that people tend to assume that what happens in the world must always have meaning and significance. These assumptions are shattered and require restoration in the event of illness, loss, or trauma (Janoff-Bulman, 1992). It is paramount for the individual to exercise caution, and for the professional to help them avoid the slippery slope of descending into unrealistic pessimism after relinquishing unrealistic optimism: learnt helplessness, severe depression and anxiety, self-destructive behaviour, or excessive blaming of others. In psychology, several concepts have recently emerged that offer an alternative to victim-blaming as a means of restoring balance (Neff, 2003; Tangney et al., 2007). These approaches are rooted in positive psychology and do not focus on finding fault with the past behaviours of individuals who are troubled, ill, or traumatised. Instead, they aim to identify ways and resources to restore or enhance a person's state of equilibrium. The first level of coping that leads to this equilibrium is outlined by the theory of *resilience* (Bonanno, 2004). The next level, which addresses coping with adverse life events, is explained by the theory of *post-traumatic growth* (Tedeschi & Calhoun, 1996, 2004). This theory suggests that individuals who have experienced trauma not only manage the stressor but also undergo significant positive changes in their thinking and their relationships with the world and themselves. Notable examples of this phenomenon can be found in the work of renowned authors like Viktor Frankl (1946/2021), who drew upon his traumatic experiences in a concentration camp during the Second World War as a basis for influential psychological theories and practices. Additionally, in more ordinary cases, we can observe how the experience of a serious illness can transform an individual's values and lifestyle (Tedeschi et al., 2020).

In recent decades, post-traumatic growth has emerged as a highly popular topic in research, garnering significant attention in public discourse. A plethora of studies have been conducted with survivors of severe trauma and illness, and it has been demonstrated that many have become more accepting, adaptable, and patient and have a better appreciation of life after illness (Barskova & Oesterreich, 2009; Hefferon et al., 2009). Furthermore, numerous individuals reported an enhanced capacity to cope with the stress of the illness, the ability to live in the present, a diminished longing for lost opportunities of the past or promises of the future, and a heightened appreciation of the support they received from their environment

(Tedeschi et al., 2020). For many, these experiences led to a re-evaluation of what they considered important in life and an increased openness to spiritual and existential values. The positive effects observed have been associated with faster recovery, less anxiety, and an improved quality of life. However, it remains unclear which factor influences the other: does post-traumatic growth promote recovery, or does enhanced physical and mental well-being lead to more positive attitudes? Additionally, another question arises: is the principle of post-traumatic growth applicable to all individuals? As the philosopher Nietzsche (1888/2009) suggested in his autobiography *Ecce homo*, those who have previously demonstrated effective coping strategies may benefit from adversity. Consequently, the applicability of the aphorism 'What does not kill him makes him stronger' may be limited. In contrast to Nietzsche's original idea, this aphorism has become commonplace in public discourse over time, quoted by filmmakers, writers, musicians, politicians, and everyday people alike. This is confirmed by the literature on the popularisation of science in psychology, which often explicitly implies the message in the title of professional and popular psychology books (Joseph, 2013). For many, this message may serve as a source of positive motivation and affirmation. However, for others, it may reinforce feelings of insecurity, anxiety, self-deprecation, and self-doubt if they feel unable to live up to this expectation (Infurna & Jayawickreme, 2021). Excessive expectations can foster the illusion of post-traumatic growth, a self-protective distortion employed to cope with the stress associated with changes in self-image and the loss of coherence caused by illness, trauma, or anxiety (Cheng et al., 2020; Ho & Cheng, 2023). It is also possible that the two types of growth represent two stages of a process. The illusory, self-protective change is more short term and occurs along with the initial challenges of coping with stress and anxiety. In contrast, the fundamental attitude change is characterised by the long-term stage (Tedeschi et al., 2018; Whitney & Taku, 2023).

In summary, it is important to note that, by definition, post-traumatic growth following an illness is anticipated if the individual concerned perceives the illness as trauma (Marziliano et al., 2024). Unfortunately, this aspect is often neglected by both professionals and non-experts, leading to a range of issues such as a desire for post-traumatic growth, illusory growth, self-blame, or even the blaming of patients due to a poorly understood set of expectations (Panchuk, 2024). These feelings may also be associated with health anxiety, which can further contribute to misconceptions and maladaptive health behaviours. Conversely, the concept of trauma is now considerably diluted and overused. In public discourse, the term is often utilised to describe everyday stressful situations and emotional strains, much like other simplistic explanations such as the claim that stress causes cancer (Ma & Kroemer, 2024). These simplifications may also aim to reduce anxiety and the need to seek safety and control. It is also important to recognise that, while the concept of post-traumatic growth seems to be universally valid, its practical application may be influenced by assumptions rooted in Western, individualistic societies (Splevins et al., 2010).

'Bio-morality' and the 'wellness syndrome'

The quest for safety and control in health and illness is complex because the start of a disease is often unclear. People find it difficult to pinpoint when their body first began to act abnormally, a challenge made worse by modern diagnostics that can detect disease before symptoms appear, often only identifiable by machines. AI has advanced to a level where it can sometimes identify bodily changes more accurately than specialists (Alowais et al., 2023; McKinney et al., 2020; Quinn et al., 2021; Younis et al., 2024). This suggests that uncertainty in human knowledge complicates the definition of boundaries between health and disease and the decision on when to intervene. The bio-psycho-social approach promotes a 'wellness continuum', making it difficult to determine when illness begins or when a person is 'completely well'. The process of pathologising risk – perceiving actions that threaten health as abnormal and reacting strongly – is linked to the process of pathologising life, labelling more sensations and behaviours as abnormal. For example, many children once called 'lively' are now diagnosed with attention deficit hyperactivity disorder (ADHD), labelled 'hyperactive', and often medicated (Klasen, 2000). Similarly, premenstrual symptoms have been categorised as 'premenstrual syndrome' (PMS), and several drugs are available to alleviate them. Through this medicalising approach, prevention also takes on the role of a 'cure', suggesting that complete health is unattainable. From this perspective, it is challenging to ascertain whether an individual's unhealthy condition can justify a lack of attention to their body and the continual neglect of various health practices. Moreover, it raises questions about the limits of personal responsibility and may also evoke feelings of guilt and anxiety. For many, this approach may suggest that self-mastery is the sole condition for health, implying that illness results from the self's failure to care for itself.

According to the classical concept of the sick role, health and illness are partly motivational issues (Parsons, 1951). This means that for a person exhibiting symptoms to be deemed socially ill, they must adopt the sick role, which involves perceiving oneself as needing assistance or treatment. According to this traditional theory, the sick role includes both the helping role and the authority of the professional, relieving the patient of specific social obligations. However, if the patient's role also includes the responsibility to improve their health, then extending this idea to the whole continuum of wellness, it can be said that the individual must also take action to maintain their health and continually improve and perfect it. This leads us back to the same circular reasoning: the individual's concern for their health, even when trapped in a vicious cycle, is related to the boundaries of health and illness, as well as questions of personal agency and responsibility. This is particularly relevant, given that the original sick role theory was developed in the 1950s. Since then, there has been a notable shift in the democratisation of healthcare, with patients being empowered and held accountable.

In critical social theory, the concept of *bio-morality* emerged partly as a result of evaluating these developments (Omelichkin, 2020). This concept posits that many people increasingly perceive negativity, lack, disappointment, and unhappiness as moral failings. As the Slovenian philosopher Slavoj Žižek notes, this phenomenon is also connected to the fact that contemporary culture is characterised by pleasure seeking at the behest of the Superego (Žižek, 2002). In other words, it is not the punitive, paternalistic Superego that drives this behaviour, but rather one that promotes self-fulfilment and pleasure. According to Žižek, there is a paradoxical relationship between enjoyment and guilt. As a person experiences more pleasure, they may feel more guilty and anxious. This sense of guilt stems from uncertainty about whether the individual is following their inner desires or simply obeying external pressure to prioritise their wellness. As Žižek stated, the emerging postmodern Superego is not restrictive in that it does not forbid us from doing things. Instead, it urges us to do more. However, it is inherently unsatisfied and perpetually frustrated with our actions. The message it conveys is that perfect pleasure is unattainable, and genuine pleasure cannot be achieved at will.

In examining the contradictions of self-care, some authors have identified a phenomenon known as *wellness syndrome* (Cederström & Spicer, 2015). Symptoms of wellness syndrome may include anxiety, self-blame, and guilt, which stem from the fact that self-care is no longer merely a personal choice but has transformed into a societal expectation due to the influence of consumer culture. This expectation can be viewed as an imposition, as it overlooks social and individual differences (Kaplan, 2019). This can also result in a kind of passive nihilism, as people's inability to comply with the perceived or absolute command of self-fulfilment can generate severe frustration and anxiety. In contemporary Western culture, where narcissism is increasingly prevalent, individuals may even develop punitive self-hatred as a result (Cederström & Spicer, 2015; Lasch, 1979). This occurs because of the compulsion to strive for narcissistic self-perfection. The individual is driven by the hidden message that their future, potential self is more important than their present self. They focus on what they can become rather than who they are. The extensive range of available options can also give rise to anxiety, as the individual may feel overwhelmed by the number of potential selves they could be. While having the freedom to choose is beneficial, it can also lead to feelings of guilt and anxiety when biological or social factors beyond their control prevent them from achieving their desired outcome. Notably, in welfare societies that emphasise autonomy and self-care, this can lead to a high risk of victim-blaming (Gunderman, 2000). Lifestyle and fashion magazines and websites often cite the aphorism attributed to George Orwell that 'At fifty, everyone has the face they deserve', while hiding the underlying messages from cosmetics companies that generate advertising revenue, especially for women. These messages suggest that if we are not careful, our past behaviours and 'mistakes' will be visible on our faces, tempting others with the idea that those who look after themselves properly can hide the signs of ageing.

As discussed in various sections of this volume, individuals preoccupied with monitoring, controlling, and improving their bodies and health are not only self-focused but also tend to compare themselves with others. This can lead to increased anxiety and guilt, along with negative, blaming attitudes towards those less concerned with health. Those who perceive negative attitudes and aim to avoid marginalisation will engage in diverse forms of self-improvement, including diet, exercise, happiness training, coaching, and meditation. They do so in line with the suggestions of their environment, beliefs, and Superego, regarding achieving perfect health and well-being. Moreover, the moral expectations surrounding personal health and overall physical and mental well-being may have contributed to a shift in the perception of the ideal employee in some companies. As Cederström and Spicer (2015) argue, instead of being a workaholic, the preferred employee might now be someone passionate about exercise. A growing number of companies are implementing comprehensive wellness programmes that encompass the entire individual. These initiatives involve ongoing monitoring of employee health, including dietary habits, sleep patterns, and other lifestyle factors (Nopper & Zelickson, 2023). While some individuals regard close monitoring as an invasion of privacy, many employees recognise it as a beneficial measure. They understand that maintaining good health not only enhances their well-being but also positively affects their professional reputation. Of course, companies cannot force healthy lifestyles upon their employees; they can only encourage and support them in making healthy choices. However, a lingering question remains regarding how effectively companies can demonstrate, in a professional and scientifically valid manner – without inducing guilt or anxiety – which behaviours are truly beneficial for health (Daniels et al., 2021).

Conclusion

When discussing responsibility and blame concerning health and illness, focusing only on an individual's behaviour while ignoring their context can lead to victim-blaming and diminish their sense of agency and autonomy. A belief in a just world may cause people to attribute the causes of illness to the patient's behaviour or lifestyle choices. However, disease or trauma can also provide new insights through resilience and post-traumatic growth. Critically examining contemporary narratives and public discourses around post-traumatic growth can also reveal how these might set both explicit and implicit expectations for patients. Feelings of inadequacy and self-blame are not unique to illness. However, they are also linked to other phenomena within our culture, where the pursuit of happiness and pleasure might generate guilt and contribute to health inequalities. An important aspect of the 'wellness syndrome' is that, amid widespread uncertainty and contradictions about the vast array of information concerning the body, health, and illness, it is relatively easy to reinforce the implicit message that those who do not prioritise their physical well-being are responsible. As the boundaries of fitness, health, and well-being become increasingly blurred and adaptable, there is a growing sense of uncertainty about one's fitness levels, dissatisfaction with one's performance, and ongoing self-criticism. This fosters a constant feeling of anxiety and guilt, which can have long-term adverse effects on health. Therefore, it is vital to recognise the complex interconnections between these factors and to develop effective strategies, both individually and collectively, to challenge dominant cultural narratives and better manage the complex dynamics between them.

7

DILEMMAS OF BODY POSITIVITY AND HEALTH CONCERNS

Body image is a significant aspect of physical and mental well-being. A vital question in fostering a healthy and anxiety-free approach to one's body and a sense of safety is whether body image is defined by positive self-acceptance or by negative attitudes, rejection, or devaluation. Previous research has predominantly focused on the relationship between negative body image, associated anxiety, and problematic behaviour or illness, as well as the devaluation and rejection of the body (Tylka & Wood-Barcalow, 2015). Negative body image is associated with adverse outcomes, including eating disorders, depression, negative emotions, social anxiety, lack of confidence, and risk behaviour, indicating lower psychological well-being (Avalos et al., 2005). In recent decades, critical social and health scientists, psychotherapists, and other professionals have observed a growing sense of ambivalence and disengagement towards the body (Orbach, 2010; Romeo, 2020). This trend has been accompanied by an increase in anxiety, rejection, and dissatisfaction, particularly due to the influence of social media. The urgency to address this issue is becoming more pronounced today. Nevertheless, conventional body image therapies, which frequently take a clinical and medicalised approach, are viewed as being insufficient for fostering a positive body image (Markula et al., 2008). Moreover, there is an increasing demand for psychology to focus not only on the cognitive aspects of body image but also on subjective experiences and the lived processes of the body (Tylka & Piran, 2019).

Framing positive body image

As positive psychology is a relatively new approach, most practitioners have not previously sought to identify correlations between body image, well-being, and

DOI: 10.4324/9781003517788-7

happiness. Instead, they have concentrated on the tensions and symptoms that arise from the debates about the appearance, the fear of ageing, the contradictions of the health cult, and how these are shaped by consumer society, globalised media culture, and society in general. All these factors contribute to distress related to the body (Featherstone et al., 1991; Milton et al., 2021). Research on the relationship between positive body image and physical and mental well-being began in the early 2000s, with a definition of positive body image emerging by the end of the decade. The three main objectives were: (1) to investigate the factors that influence the development of positive body image; (2) to explore body image characteristics that promote successful adjustment and their relationship to psychological functioning and quality of life; and (3) to develop and demonstrate practices that promote positive body image (Cash, 2004; Wood-Barcalow et al., 2010). Several dimensions of positive body image have been identified: (1) acceptance and positive appreciation of one's body's attributes (age, shape, aesthetics) and functioning (health, strength, dexterity); (2) awareness and attention to bodily experiences and needs; and (3) positive attitudes and openness to perceive and process messages from one's body and the outside world, without rejection or avoidance (Menzel & Levine, 2011).

These objectives are generally agreeable; however, achieving a positive body image in today's society – with its expectations and biases – remains uncertain. Not everyone can easily love their body regardless of shape or size. Frustration from unmet expectations can lead to anxiety, guilt, and negative health effects (Merino et al., 2024). Research indicates that acceptance and respect for the body are increasing (Tylka & Piran, 2019). These findings emphasise the importance of integrating the body and self as central to a positive body image – a state of confidence and safety where one feels at harmony with their body, expressing individuality while navigating social challenges.

Positive body image encompasses both satisfaction and positive attitudes, evaluations, and emotions towards the self. Scientific evidence suggests that positive and negative body images operate independently, exerting distinct effects on feelings, thoughts, and behaviour (Burychka et al., 2021; Gillen, 2015). This implies they are neither opposites nor extremes of the same spectrum. Positive and negative body image distinctions are determined not by overall satisfaction with one's physical appearance, but by the acceptance of the body in its current state. Negative body image involves rejection of one's physical self, leading to adverse outcomes like anxiety, avoidance behaviour, constant comparisons with others, and lack of self-confidence. Such individuals may engage in unhealthy behaviours like forced exercise, dieting, cosmetic surgery, addictions, self-harm, and self-destruction. Of course, it is possible to transform a negative body image into a positive one. However, the fact that positive and negative body images are not on the same dimension shows that this is not just a quantitative change but a qualitative one. This also explains why changes in body image during individual development affect many other aspects of identity and behaviour (Tort-Nasarre et al., 2023). A notable phenomenon is the gendered aspect of this, along with the societal changes that have resulted in men experiencing more anxiety about their appearance than before (Piatkowski et al., 2024).

An illustrative example of successful positive body image development is that of the young Australian woman with Down syndrome, Madeleine Stuart. Ms Stuart first graced the runway at New York Fashion Week in 2015 at the age of 16 and has since become a luminary on catwalks around the globe. She has garnered a significant following on social media and has been featured in numerous articles, photographs, and magazine covers. She was also the subject of a feature-length documentary, *Maddy the Model* (Magnusson, 2020). This film raises questions about the balance between her ambition and her mother's influence. Nevertheless, Maddy would not have achieved her goals without consistent support. Favourable external evaluations and appreciation of the body significantly bolster a positive body image and self-acceptance. Research indicates that a positive body image is directly linked to personality traits such as optimism, positive emotions, self-esteem, life satisfaction, and happiness. It demonstrates that body image is associated with self-confidence and elevated self-esteem (Tylka, 2011). However, research on well-being and body image has primarily concentrated on hedonic well-being, emphasising positive emotions, happiness, and a positive self-image (Swami et al., 2018). It is increasingly argued that a perspective considering both hedonic (emotional) and eudaimonic (self-actualising) well-being is necessary to understand the relationship between body image and subjective well-being. This holistic model clarifies that a positive body image can contribute to positive emotional states, self-actualisation, personality development, and social relationships. Extending this research to children, where the focus has primarily been on negative body image and its detrimental consequences, may be particularly beneficial by focusing on fostering body awareness and self-acceptance (Halliwell et al., 2017; Maes et al., 2021).

From body positivity to body neutrality

The growing visibility of this topic in public discourse and media suggests that body image is no longer an issue confined to academia; instead, it has evolved into a concern for the public. Recent examples of body-positive movements exemplify this aim, which strives to ensure that all bodies, regardless of their characteristics or condition, receive the same acceptance and respect.

Protest movements against societal ideals of beauty and the normative appearance expected by society have emerged since the late 19th century, often linked to various waves of feminist movements (Butler, 1993). A recent development is that the movement has transcended feminist rhetoric and evolved into a significant civil forum and activism, mainly through social media (Riley et al., 2019).

The precursor to the body-positive movement was initiated in the United States in 1996 (Sobczak, 2014). The initiative's primary objective was to challenge the body ideals perpetuated by the media, which are often inaccessible to many individuals. Additionally, the initiative aimed to reduce the prevalence of eating disorders, self-image problems, and low self-esteem among women and men by promoting the acceptance and beauty of bodies of all shapes, ages, and colours. The term 'body positivity' first appeared in 2010 on the Australian online site *Female for Life* (Montgomery, 2010). The movement has been mainly boosted by its strong presence on Instagram since 2012. Social media has regularly depicted women as heroines by showcasing their struggles with eating disorders, opposing those who stigmatise non-conforming body features, and challenging the 'bikini body' myth and postpartum body ideals through unedited photos. However, most content still portrays idealised female bodies (Chowdhury et al., 2025; Rodgers et al., 2024).

However, the question arises as to how 'unretouched' a photo can be, and how unvarnished it can be in showing the reality of the body. This is particularly poignant today, as the combination of digitisation and social media usage has led to the emergence of new medicalised concepts in popular discourse such as 'Zoom dysmorphia' or 'Snapchat dysmorphia' (Ramphul, 2022; Ramphul & Meijas, 2018). The French philosopher and essayist Roland Barthes argues that the camera lens does not directly depict reality as it is, but instead records a version of past reality (Barthes, 2000). This encompasses the common understanding of the medium, particularly from the photographer's perspective, and influences how different cultures perceive the portrayal of the body and photography. As a result, even the most seemingly natural photograph reveals more than just the objective truth of the body, as the photographer often unintentionally aims to express more than what is immediately visible. It also contains multiple layers of meaning and both conscious and unconscious messages.

Adherents of the body-positive movement have become increasingly vocal about the fundamental goal of challenging societal ideals about the body; anxiety-provoking, unrealistic expectations; and enhancing self-acceptance and self-worth by improving self-image through the realisation of a love of one's own body (Ladwig et al., 2024; Rodgers et al., 2022). The movement emphasises its support for all those who fall outside beauty norms. This self-definition closely aligns with the concept of a positive body image, with almost identical objectives. The body-positive movement gained such popularity that by 2022, there were around 18 million posts featuring the hashtag 'bodypositive' (Clark, 2022). Consequently, fashion and beauty companies have been compelled to reduce the extent of retouching in their images and to consider consumer demands regarding body size (Tsawaab, 2023). The initiative has been a resounding success. However, some dissenting voices have seen the campaign as a business gimmick and failed to recognise its importance for body image, self-acceptance, and health (Stamp, 2019). Moreover, there is an increasing amount of research on commercialising the body positivity movement and utilising Instagram as an advertising platform for sharing key messages related to body positivity (Cwynar-Horta, 2016). Many fashion brands now advertise themselves as 'body positive' and question whether they can be so even if they only feature make-up-free or plus-size models in their collections. This is supported by the fact that PR firms seek out influencers to help them create their profiles and, of course, to be seen in products belonging to the brand (Brewster & Sklar, 2022). Conversely, there are also examples of high-quality campaigns and educational support programmes on body acceptance. For instance, a few years ago, the Disney animated short film *Reflect* was expected to have a positive impact (Lock, 2022). The film follows the journey of a plus-sized ballet dancer named Bianca as she grapples with self-doubt and body image issues. It culminates in her self-acceptance and regaining her charm and strength. In the meantime, however, there have been public debates in the international press about whether the portrayal of a protagonist with a less-than-ideal body is affirming for children or whether it can harm their physical and psychological development by 'propagating' obesity (Berlin, 2022). However, such films are urgently needed because, for instance, a study of 180 children's cartoons found that 87% of female characters were portrayed as underweight, unwittingly illustrating an 'ideal' body type and an implicit bias against the overweight (Northup & Liebler, 2010).

While body-positive movements have had several beneficial effects, their focus on the aesthetic dimensions of the body, even if it emphasises acceptance, can be seen as a limitation. The internal instability of the movement is also indicated by the recent publication of books by authors who were initially ardent proponents of body positivity but who found it problematic that the struggle against marginalisation and oppression, which is otherwise a vital mission of the body positivity movement, leaves less room for genuine acceptance of the body (Kneeland, 2023). Others recognise that the external expectation to always love one's body and to not openly express changing emotions is limiting, sometimes even causing anxiety (Meyers, 2023). This may even be the starting point for health anxiety.

The effect of body positivity expectations on health anxiety is complex, with recent research showing both positive and negative effects. Positive body image enhances self-esteem and reduces body dissatisfaction, greatly lowering general anxiety, depression, and health-related anxiety (Cohen et al., 2019). Additionally, body positivity builds resilience against the media's unrealistic portrayals of beauty and health, as well as resistance to incorporating harmful body images (Tiggemann & McGill, 2004). In terms of negative affectivity, research has shown that concerns about body image have been significantly associated with health anxiety in both clinical and non-clinical samples (Rodgers et al., 2023). This may be due to the underlying process of hypervigilance, where individuals with negative body image are often cautious about changes in their appearance and bodily sensations. This can lead to a bias towards health-related information, which in turn increases health anxiety. Conversely, catastrophic thinking, which is also closely linked to negative body image, can influence individuals to see even minor health issues as signs of serious illness (Seto & Nakao, 2017). It is also important to mention the phenomenon of *inauthentic positivity*. This is the effect of expectations that result in superficial, contrived expressions of positivity and the hiding of problems, such as health concerns, for which the person cannot access support and help, thereby worsening the problem (Cramblitt & Pritchard, 2013). This can be especially dangerous if concerns about genuine health issues do not arise, leaving the condition unnoticed and potentially leading to serious consequences from late medical intervention.

Initiatives have been introduced to address these body positivity issues and are gaining traction, spearheading the 'body neutrality' movement. In their analysis of over 100 related websites, Pellizzer and Wade (2023) identified three main characteristics of body neutrality. First, they argue that body neutrality implies a realistic, flexible, and neutral attitude towards the body. Second, it values and promotes the body's functionality, and third, the basis for evaluating oneself is not one's appearance. Of these, functionality is particularly important for maintaining a positive body image and promoting health and well-being (Alleva & Tylka, 2021). The body neutrality movement encourages individuals to shift their focus from appearance to body functionality and health. This shift can help to reduce the anxiety that is commonly experienced because of societal pressures to maintain a particular body image. By emphasising what the body, whether male or female, can achieve rather than its appearance, individuals may gain a greater control over their bodies and experience a reduction in health anxiety. Recent studies suggest that adopting a body neutrality perspective can lower body dissatisfaction and related anxiety (Clark, 2022). Body neutrality may promote a more balanced approach to health, emphasising overall well-being rather than striving for an ideal body shape. This perspective can reduce the obsessive behaviours often seen in health anxiety, such as excessive checking of physical symptoms or constant comparison with others.

These are encouraging results, and some scholars argue that the body neutrality construct has features common with body positivity (Wood-Barcalow et al., 2024). Still, it remains to be seen to what extent body neutrality can ensure that feelings are experienced and do not take us in a more emotion-free direction (Tiggemann, 2024). A lack of emotional attachment can initially lead to body-related anxieties and self-destructive behaviours. While interventions to neutralise negative body image may reduce harmful thoughts and behaviours, they could also distract from self-care and recognising dysfunctional signals (Hefferon, 2015). Although body neutrality aims to decrease appearance-based anxiety, some might perceive it as neglecting their body and health, thereby risking the neglect of important health behaviours and screenings.

Healthy at every size?

Whether focusing on body neutrality or positivity is the most effective approach to improving health outcomes remains a question. In addition to acknowledging the benefits and social importance of body positivity for physical and mental health, critics have also highlighted the potential for accepting all body sizes, even with conditions such as anorexia or obesity, to undermine the successes that professionals have achieved in the fight against disease in recent decades (McWhorter, 2020).

The social and ethical dilemmas surrounding the unrestricted acceptance and public display of bodies in any shape and condition, alongside the complex issues of artistic freedom, personal autonomy, and health, are sharply exemplified in the case of Norwegian photographer Lene Marie Fossen, whose story is depicted in the shockingly beautiful documentary *Self-Portrait* (Høgset et al., 2020). Fossen, who determined at the age of 10 that she wished to remain a child and refused to eat, suffered from severe anorexia, rejected treatment, and dramatically portrayed her emaciated body in her artistic works until her death at the age of 33, gaining international acclaim and provoking profound debates (Pawlak, 2022).

As for obesity, opponents of the body-positive movement have noted that the proportion of overweight people in the global population has tripled in the last 50 years (McWhorter, 2020). The approach of treating obesity as a chronic disease has helped to reduce health risks. However, this approach has focused on medical solutions rather than addressing social and environmental factors such as health literacy deficits, inequalities in the availability of healthy food, and the substantial influence of the food industry, including the promotion of junk food. It is also important to note that critical social science approaches view the medicalisation of obesity as a social construct and point to a gap between public health concerns and individual life situations, as well as concerns and opportunities for change (Ferreira & Webber, 2023). This is supported, for example, by Natalie Boero (2012), who found that overweight individuals often seek weight loss not primarily for health reasons but also to fit into society and escape stigma. She also discussed how the media plays a significant role in shaping the obesity 'epidemic' and associated panic. Boero argues that movements such as Body Positive and Health at Every Size (HAES) provide essential insights into how social issues shape our understanding of body image, as well as concepts of health, illness, and normality.

Additionally, some strands of body-positive rhetoric portray overweight individuals as victims and view obesity as a human right (Morris, 2019). In other conceptualisations, obesity can be seen as an addiction, especially if related to food addiction (Rogers & Smit, 2020). Following this thought, consumer society and food industry can also be held accountable (Ferreira & Webber, 2023). At this juncture, it becomes pertinent to inquire whether the acceptance of severe obesity does not also signify an endorsement of its health risks. This is of practical consequence, given the publication of popular educational materials that explicitly proclaim being overweight is not a health risk (Bacon, 2010). Some critics have argued that the body-positive movement, by encouraging excessive self-acceptance, may devalue health-promoting behaviour and reinforce risk behaviour (McWhorter, 2020). Furthermore, some see obesity as solely the individual's responsibility (and fault), arguing that the rest of society should not bear the additional health costs (Muttarak, 2018; Robinson et al., 2017).

An example of the overarching dilemmas and complex contradictions that this issue raises can be seen in the debate that arose in 2007 following an article by a British epidemiologist (Roberts, 2007). The article suggested that reducing obesity could help combat global warming, a topic that has significantly impacted and continues to captivate the scientific community. Roberts argued that overweight individuals consume more food, increasing carbon emissions. This perspective understandably sparked debate, with concerns expressed about further stigmatisation of overweight individuals and heightened body and health anxiety. Body-positive activists and other critics argued that this system of scapegoating is a moral attack on a huge group of people (Byniarski & Brock, 2022). The debate remains open and has been revisited in various scientific journals (Villarroya & Giralt, 2024). For example, an article published in *Obesity*, the official journal of The Obesity Society and a premier source of scientific information, concluded that an overweight person contributes 20% more greenhouse gas emissions than a person of 'normal' body mass (Magkos et al., 2020). However, research that highlights the inverse correlation has also been published, suggesting that global warming may contribute to obesity (Kanazawa, 2019). Additionally, there has been considerable recent attention to the possibility that global warming may contribute to childhood obesity, for instance, by preventing parents from allowing children to exercise outdoors on extremely hot summer days (Morrison, 2022).

The links, therefore, are at least two-way, and blaming and stigmatising those involved are not the way forward. Furthermore, the stigmatisation of overweight individuals is concerning, as obesity poses a health problem that is at least as significant as malnutrition (Chong et al., 2023). Obesity has been linked to a range of chronic diseases such as type 2 diabetes, hypertension, stroke, and several cancers (Riaz et al., 2023). Furthermore, the debate has intensified over the past 15 to 20 years concerning how being overweight has predominantly been framed within medical discourse. This has fostered anxieties due to the singular focus on individual responsibility in presenting this as a medical issue (Murray, 2008; Rathbone et al., 2023). Research in the early 2000s demonstrated that mentions of individual responsibility ranged from 72% to 98%, with no regard for the social context. At the same time, in scientific communications, the proportion was approximately 40% (Saguy & Almeling, 2008). Weight stigma in media content remains widespread and harmful, yet there is a lack of guidance on how to reduce it (Kite et al., 2022). For example, recent studies have shown that UK newspaper coverage of obesity often uses fear-inducing rhetoric, blaming individuals within neoliberal discourses. Media and health texts employ these tactics to attract attention and encourage compliance with recommendations (Brookes & Baker, 2021). A dichotomy also emerged in the discourse, creating 'alarmist' and 'sceptical' counter-camps (Robinson, 2017; Rathbone et al., 2023.). Sceptics argue that diet and exercise should be based on individual needs and well-being, not body size.

Alarmists warn that ignoring scientific evidence – that obesity increases health risks and weight loss is beneficial – perpetuates health and economic issues. Opponents advocate accepting body size and intuitive eating, warning that restrictive diets can cause distress (Hazzard et al., 2021; Outland, 2010). A demonstration of this is that women's acceptance of their bodies is less reliant on their body mass index (BMI) index and more influenced by feedback from their social environment (Ahadzadeh et al., 2018).

All these debates likely contributed to recent recommendations by the Lancet Commission for the clinical diagnosis of obesity, which do not include BMI but instead focus on the degree of adiposity (Rubino et al., 2025). Body-positive groups promoting body acceptance and intuitive eating saw improvements in self-esteem and reduced obesity prejudice (Humphrey et al., 2015). Reducing stigma is advantageous as it can sometimes be more detrimental than overweight itself. A debate persists regarding whether the acceptance of one's weight enhances mental health and, by extension, physical health. The February 2021 issue of *Cosmopolitan* magazine used the slogan 'This is Healthy!' to promote body diversity, supported by 11 interviews. Critics expressed concerns that emphasising the overweight condition, particularly during the COVID-19 pandemic, could pose risks, given that excess weight is a recognised risk factor for the virus (Preskey, 2021). Conversely, some contend that messages of self-acceptance are essential for mental health during crises, as many individuals experience anxiety and insecurity (Monaghan et al., 2022; Salles, 2021). This discussion prompts critical questions regarding the definition of health, personal responsibility, and empowerment – concepts often portrayed in conflicting ways within the media, which subsequently influence health behaviours and access to healthcare based on attitudes towards body image.

Body dissatisfaction and health inequalities

There is a strong correlation between body appreciation and several factors related to physical and mental well-being, including self-esteem, self-compassion, and sexual satisfaction (Linardon et al., 2022). These have been studied more extensively in the context of mental health, whereas their impact on physical health and disease has been less explored. However, it can be assumed that negative body image and lower levels of body appreciation contribute to more hidden patterns of health anxiety and distress. Negative attitudes and devaluation of the body, especially weight stigma, are substantial causes of health inequality (Albert et al., 2024); they are associated with decreased help-seeking behaviour, a lack of communication of symptoms, or less frequent use of health services. For example, research shows a correlation between lower body appreciation and higher self-criticism levels among Romanian university students, as well as poorer oral health status and inadequate oral health behaviour (Dumitrescu et al., 2014). This is also consistent with the findings among young people with psoriasis, where perceived stigma associated with the disease was more pronounced among those with higher body weight

(Mazurkiewicz et al., 2021). The result is noteworthy because, in this group, they otherwise rated their health status as good. A recent review found that body dissatisfaction may be a barrier to health behaviours regarding screening attendance (Goh et al., 2024); here, attendance at screening was more strongly associated with overall satisfaction with appearance than with satisfaction with specific body parts. The exception to this was skin cancer screening, which may be explained by the fact that it is not limited to a specific body area/part. At the same time, there was also some correlation with satisfaction with body parts. For example, women who were more satisfied with their genitals were more likely to have a gynaecological check-up, and women who were more satisfied with the size of their breasts were more likely to have a self-check-up (Goh et al., 2024). It is important to note, however, that these studies have tended to be conducted among young women, and there is less data on the relationship between breast satisfaction and preventive health behaviours among older women. In contrast to younger women, older women are less likely to engage in gynaecological screening. In a previous study, Ridolfi and Crowther (2013) suggested that body shaming and body avoidance significantly influence women's participation in screenings. They hypothesised that self-efficacy, health anxiety, risk perception, and subjective norms play a role.

In light of these considerations, it is imperative to conduct comprehensive research on these factors, incorporating not only body satisfaction and age but also health literacy factors and the role of cultural attitudes and expectations regarding women's bodies as they age. Research suggests that the importance of appearance is more pronounced among women and that men are less likely to attend screening tests than women (Quittkat et al., 2019). Similarly, more attention should be paid to the associations between child and adolescent body image and health behaviours beyond aspects related to body weight. One Norwegian study found a correlation between body dissatisfaction and poor health status ratings among adolescents aged 11–15 years (Meland et al., 2007). At the same time, it should also be considered that lower self-esteem affects the entire physical and psychological spectrum. One's perception of poorer health may not be associated with increased preventive health behaviour, but rather with increased risk behaviour due to increased anxiety and self-neglect arising from low self-esteem.

Biased bodies in healthcare

Health professionals are pivotal in shaping individuals' relationships with their bodies. However, they must also be aware of the sources of information and media influences on the general public. One of the most significant functions of body-positive websites is that they aim to provide a safe space for personal narratives and images of bodies that are not considered ideal. Furthermore, the movement has witnessed the emergence of online platforms like #Diagnosisfat# where individuals share their personal experiences and narratives of discrimination and mistreatment within the healthcare sector (Goldware, 2022). It is important to acknowledge that these reports are subjective, and the views of health professionals remain uncertain. Nevertheless, the patients felt stigmatised, which impacted their quality of life and their relationships with healthcare providers. It is also evident that the attitudes of health professionals can significantly influence their perceptions of the physical characteristics of the clients (Mohamed et al., 2016).

Recent research has found that weight stigma can hinder healthcare access and utilisation (Pearl & Sheynblyum, 2025). An earlier survey of policymakers in 10 developed countries worldwide on healthcare biases revealed that the majority, 90%, identified a lack of personal motivation as a major cause of obesity (Cooper, 2014). The individualisation of the problem and the stigmatisation of those affected were strongly emphasised. The stigmatisation of overweight individuals is not a novel phenomenon. Rather, it can be argued that this attitude itself constitutes a significant public health problem. Consequently, the adverse effects at the individual level are not separate from the social anxieties produced by medical, political, and media discourse, including even seemingly benevolent educational practices and public health strategies (Monaghan et al., 2022). A recent study employing a qualitative methodology revealed that the theme of body image was inadequately represented in the discourse among health practitioners (Sharp et al., 2023). However, they acknowledged that the body-positive movement could influence their practice. The concept of body neutrality was relatively unknown, yet it was preferred over body positivity. The latter was also recognised as necessary, but its perceived 'promotion' of obesity and connection to the pro-anorexia movement was viewed as harmful.

Several studies have reported an overweight bias among health professionals and university students, including physiotherapists and nutritionists (Panza et al., 2018). In an earlier study of trainee dietitians, doctors, nurses, and nutritionists in the UK, the prevalence of fat phobia was found to be alarmingly high, with only 1.4% of respondents exhibiting a positive attitude (Swift et al., 2013). Negative attitudes and reported frustration with the treatment of overweight patients were also present among Canadian general practitioners (GPs) (Alberga et al., 2019). This was particularly the case among male doctors. Similar attitudes have been reported in other studies. For instance, some GPs believed that overweight patients were less cooperative, and physicians felt less useful in counselling them, making it less likely that they would be engaged by professionals (Jay et al., 2009). In an extensive survey of six countries (Australia, Canada, France, the UK, Germany, and the U.S.), two-thirds of those who experienced stigma related to their weight also experienced it from health professionals and were less likely to visit a doctor, less likely to attend screening tests, and generally had poorer health outcomes (Puhl et al., 2021).

Therefore, it is essential for health professionals to be aware of their views and attitudes and to adopt a complex, non-individualising perspective on the issue, as only in this way can they help their clients process information, develop health literacy, and provide support. This is also of particular importance because some research has found a link between body weight stigma and perceived or actual discrimination and mortality risks among Americans over 50 years (Sutin et al., 2015). This risk is similar to that associated with smoking, for example, and was not linked to actual body weight. The mediating factors behind this phenomenon are not yet clear. However, they are thought to include social isolation, lower self-care motivations, and lead to an inadequate quality of health care, which is also a mediating factor. This has been highlighted by research which found that in chronic conditions with physical limitations or disfigurations (e.g. amputations, severe wounds), professionals adopted a patronising attitude and had lower expectations of the quality of life and rehabilitation capacity and opportunities of these patients (Hrehorów et al., 2012). Furthermore, research indicates that patients who perceived stigmatisation from professionals exhibited higher anxiety, depression, and lower self-esteem (Treufeldt & Burton, 2024). Therefore, professionals must be aware of their own body image beliefs and the broader issue of body image, in general, to help clients develop a more positive, anxiety-free attitude towards their bodies and health (Talumaa et al., 2022). Despite research indicating that health professionals recognise the importance of the topic, a significant knowledge gap remains among them. This is reflected in the fact that the issue of body image is often described as 'slippery' (Lamarche et al., 2020).

The notion of 'medical gaslighting' has gained recognition in recent years within the media and public discourse. It highlights that the concerns of marginalised and physically disadvantaged groups are sometimes given less weight in healthcare (Durbhakula & Fortin, 2023). Such awareness may help to promote dialogue between professionals and laypeople. Further education and research into positive body image could improve the provider-patient relationship and, consequently, psychological well-being and overall health, while also reducing stress and health anxiety. Social science approaches that emphasise the body's role in healthcare and health behaviour are now supported by empirical evidence. Psychology is also beginning to consider factors such as age, gender, cultural aspects, healthcare communication, and the development of a positive body image. Integrating research findings into healthcare practice and raising awareness can significantly enhance positive body image and autonomy over health behaviours, as well as promote both physical and mental health.

Conclusion

This chapter has analysed the notable shift in body image research that has led to the rise of body-positive and body-neutral movements, along with the challenges in fostering positive body image and self-acceptance. The body positivity movement, as a social initiative, offers a potential approach for building confidence and security in a culture that often stigmatises diverse body types. It also raises ethical questions and concerns about individual and societal autonomy and freedom, which may conflict with health-related issues, especially for those who are excessively underweight or overweight. The influence of social media on self-perception is particularly influential in contemporary society, affecting body image and related health anxieties. Furthermore, issues such as body dissatisfaction, felt stigma, and bias in healthcare settings can create disparities in access to services and may hinder the provider-patient relationship. The perspectives of health professionals regarding the body-positive movement, body image, and their implications for clients' health behaviours warrant further research in both academic and clinical settings.

8

FINDING SAFETY IN MEANING AND CONNECTION

Globalisation, technological development, and digital culture – particularly, the rise of AI and social media – foster new values and forms of connectivity while generating significant insecurities and anxieties regarding our relationship with the body and health. Consequently, psychology faces considerable future challenges and responsibilities to provide answers and develop methods and procedures that enable personalised solutions for achieving stable physical and mental balance and a sense of safety. The following sections will critically assess contemporary dilemmas in the quest for safety through well-being, self-help, meaning-making, resonance, and connectedness.

Well-being in need of context

Well-being is a central theme in contemporary health psychology, public health, and social policy, and its significance is further emphasised by increasing social inequalities (Jackson et al., 2022). In an optimistic yet decontextualised approach, it is often regarded as a form of panacea – a condition that, if properly nurtured, could potentially mitigate inequalities. Critical and somewhat ironic interpretations have suggested that we are witnessing a 'well-being pandemic', mainly because health, well-being, and happiness often become ideological norms and expectations that create anxiety and pathologise those who fail to live up to these vague and ambiguous expectations (Jackson et al., 2022).

The formulation of a wellness model of health with a positive focus in the second half of the 20th century represented a paradigm shift, among other reasons, because when health is conceptualised as the absence of disease, it loses its inherent positive meaning (Eriksson et al., 2024; Oliver et al., 2018). However, due to

DOI: 10.4324/9781003517788-8

this paradigm shift and the early theories of positive psychology, the concept of health has overlapped mainly with ideas of subjective well-being and wellness, bio-psycho-social health, quality of life, and life satisfaction (Simons & Baldwin, 2021). Critical analysts also point out that the concept of happiness has a much more nuanced and complex set of meanings in terms of its philosophical and cultural-historical background than has been synthesised in positive psychology and used superficially in everyday discourse (Sewaybricker & Massola, 2023). A common criticism of positive psychology, which primarily addresses the topic of well-being, is that its classical authors have explicitly addressed the concepts of happiness and well-being along the axis of emotions in a quantifiable way, following a kind of neoliberal normative vision that emphasises growth and productivity (Rivera et al., 2023). These concepts should, therefore, be reinterpreted in the context of the psychopolitics of well-being, adopting a motivational approach that does not generate anxiety and guilt and is grounded in scientific evidence rather than ideological utopias (Steel et al., 2018).

A recent cross-cultural study with 66 authors has shown that the idealisation of subjective well-being and the achievement of maximum happiness, often used synonymously, is mainly a feature of 'WEIRD' (Western, Educated, Industrialised, Rich, and Democratic) countries, where people have relatively few existential burdens and a more favourable ecological habitat than in other parts of the world (Krys et al., 2024b). Analysing large-scale surveys, they conclude that the reverse is also true, that is, societies that prioritise happiness maximisation also fall into the WEIRD category. Therefore, generalising the findings of happiness and well-being research to all societies may be problematic at an ideological and political level. Similar findings are reported in a study of 63 countries and 7 sociocultural regions, which examined the cross-cultural applicability of various measures of happiness (Gardiner et al., 2020). Their results showed that the reliability of the measures was lowest in African and Middle Eastern countries and that the independent happiness schema was more coherent in WEIRD countries. The authors, who analyse geopolitical shifts in the balance of power in psychological research, also point out that in addition to the dominance of WEIRD studies, there is a tendency for cross-cultural studies to focus more on comparing Asian countries with Western countries. A review article analysing 60 cross-cultural studies and nearly one and a half million abstracts concluded that the number of articles from Confucian East Asian countries already exceeds that from Western countries, but that there is little representation of Eastern European authors and almost no representation of Pacific Island, Caribbean, Middle African, and Central Asian societies in psychological studies. As a result, messages about psychological well-being, happiness, and self-care, which, of course, reach the latter countries via the internet convey culturally alien or even inaccessible patterns and thus tend to cause frustration and anxiety in users (Krys et al., 2024a).

Partly due to these critiques, a growing view holds that both the science of well-being and its critiques are closely linked to the geopolitical features of modern consumer society (Carlisle et al., 2009; Kiknadze & Fowers, 2023). This raises questions about individual and social well-being within the context of broader global issues. The spread of consumer society influences personal well-being and is related to social phenomena such as alienation, societal fragmentation, and a diminished spiritual and ethical life. The environmental aspect, which is crucial today, heightens health concerns amid the climate crisis. Critics argue that the emphasis on individual well-being overlooks environmental factors crucial for personal experience (Watson et al., 2009). These overlooked factors can cause exploitation, harm subjective well-being, and decrease collective well-being, which ultimately also affect those in better circumstances. A further criticism is that the neoliberal concept of happiness shifts focus away from power structures by promoting self-reflection. It encourages individuals to focus only on themselves and their thoughts, rather than critically analysing social relationships. Consequently, societal suffering is privatised and psychologised (Han, 2021).

The third wave of positive psychology addresses these issues from multiple perspectives, aiming for a complex, bio-psycho-social-ecological inter- and transdisciplinary approach to well-being, thereby moving beyond disciplinary fragmentation and responding to methodological and contextual challenges (Wissing, 2022). One notable example of these conceptual shifts is the concept of resilience, which has become a central and highly successful idea in positive psychology (Luthar et al., 2000). This is particularly relevant for the arguments developed in this book because resilience has emerged as a key strategy for seeking safety and coping with anxiety. Resilience is generally viewed as a positive concept in professional and public discussions. However, in recent years, questions have arisen about whether different forms of individual resilience are beneficial in all contexts. For instance, resilience cannot be considered positive if it tolerates disparity and inequality (Suslovic & Lett, 2024). Additionally, attitudes that excuse disempowered individuals for their unhealthy behaviours can undermine their empowerment and autonomy, implying that they are not responsible for changing their lives (Mahdiani & Ungar, 2021). Studying resilience in the more advantaged, WEIRD populations obscures structural and other social and psychological issues. As noted by several authors, including Bracke (2016), many people in contemporary societies are so attached to the ideals of upward mobility, job security, and social equality that they fail to realise that these goals are unattainable for many individuals. This leads to pseudo-resilience, where they ignore the world's dangers and ecological problems. Additionally, Chandler and Reid (2016) highlight a significant issue with the concept of resilience in postmodern societies: individuals who demonstrate resilience often revert to their original circumstances after overcoming stressful events, and the fundamental social and environmental conditions that led to the initial problem remain unaddressed. Similar conflicting issues are evident in the dilemmas surrounding self-care and self-help. This raises the question of how ideas generally viewed as positive can have negative implications for equity, individual autonomy, and the overall effectiveness of health-related behaviours and safety measures.

The two faces of self-help

The emergence of the self-care approach in health behaviours in recent years is striking. In 2022, the hashtag #Selfcare received 28.2 billion views on TikTok and had 66 million posts on Instagram (Fielding, 2022). This indicates a positive attitude shift towards autonomy, control, and empowerment. However, the interpretation of self-care can vary significantly among users. On the one hand, it may involve informed and conscious health behaviours; on the other hand, it can lead to harmful consumerism fuelled by various advertising sources, both online and offline, as well as by influencers and self-proclaimed experts. As a result, self-care can encompass both positive practices and harmful habits, contributing to increased health anxiety. This concern is particularly relevant, given the proliferation of self-help literature.

Self-help literature has existed since the 18th century and emerged alongside the beginning of industrialisation. However, it gained significant popularity in the health and mental health fields during the social changes of the 1960s and the rise of mass media (Riessman & Carroll, 1995). Self-help discourse is based on a specific set of rules, which are not always transparent. However, as Michel Foucault (1988) has shown, an essential part of it is the *technologies of the self*, that is, procedures by which individuals shape, monitor, and control their behaviour, body, health, and habits according to the interests of society. To this end, self-help discourse employs specific rhetorical devices, including personal narratives, case histories, metaphors, and examples that are either appealing or discouraging (Cheng, 2007). Self-help literature and media are often presented in one of two ways. In the first approach, a knowledgeable professional provides commentary while the recipient is positioned as a passive individual in need of healing and repair, reflecting a 'wounded self' (Western, 2012). In contrast, the second approach involves the professional adopting a motivational coaching style, engaging with an active and informed audience. This audience aims to develop a 'real' or 'authentic' self. However, critical analysts have noted that self-help resources are closely tied to modern systems of power and knowledge. They often rely on moral and ethical regulation and employ the tools of governmentality (Foucault, 1988; Rimke, 2020).

The self-help genre has been the subject of considerable debate in recent decades, with interdisciplinary and critical social science perspectives examining various aspects of therapeutic culture, popular psychology, and the happiness industry (Nehring et al., 2020). As people have become inundated with self-help content, concerns have arisen about the reliability of the information, the prevalence of misleading content, and the contradictions within scientific claims. This has sparked increased criticism of the self-help movement and anxieties reflected in public discourse and the media (Schwartz, 2018; Goddard, 2024). Paradoxically, the terms 'self-help addict' and 'toxic self-help' have emerged in public discussions, often associated with works that employ pop psychology and self-help language similar to those they critique (Gefen, 2017; Lack & Rousseau, 2022). These books vary in quality and sometimes contain questionable content (Ridgway, 2017; Travers, 2022). This may be seen as a countercultural movement advocating civil action against self-improvement, consumerism, and the happiness industry or exploring alternative business solutions. Concurrently, the articles and books often convey the authors' frustrations and disillusionment, frequently referencing their decades of experience with self-help books, apps, and courses on platforms such as YouTube and TikTok, which they label as ineffective or detrimental. These authors share their personal experiences emotionally and honestly, aiming to connect with readers and foster a sense of community based on shared experiences. This approach also resonates with the overarching themes of self-help discourse (Ramage, 2005). These messages, whether from self-help literature or their opposing and alternative versions, can be unsettling for many and discourage others from seeking expert help. Carey (2020) questions how much self-help books focus on the reader versus the author when they include excessive personal experiences, stories, and anecdotes. They question the idea that 'a problem shared is a problem halved', arguing that learning from others' experiences may provide relief. Still, the resolution is for each individual to find their own relief.

When considering health anxiety and safety, it is vital to find solutions that reduce anxiety and promote effective health behaviours, encouraging proactive self-management. Bridging academic and popular psychology by presenting credible expert messages in accessible language can enhance understanding and engagement. Historically, texts from the Renaissance aimed to educate and foster culture, knowledge, and agency, helping to reduce anxiety and uncertainty (Blum, 2020). In today's world, self-help and self-improvement have evolved beyond mere psychological and moral concerns; they have also become technological issues. Numerous digital tools and technologies are available to aid in this process, as discussed in earlier chapters of this volume. As Carl Cederström and André Spicer argue in their book, *The Wellness Syndrome* (2015), the focus has shifted from simple self-improvement to continuous self-optimisation, which involves striving to meet an ideal standard. In their subsequent work, the authors describe an experiment in which they dedicated the year 2016 to various self-optimisation activities, testing different lifestyle advice (Cederström & Spicer, 2017). This critical social science fieldwork explored multiple topics, including work-related productivity, enhancing physical attractiveness, fostering creativity, and improving relationships. The authors documented their experiences in a culturally critical diary, often infused with irony. At times, however, they expressed sadness, for example when Cederström attended a retreat with a Zen guru and witnessed the suffering and desperate attempts of middle-class participants striving for self-improvement. Like other authors, Cederström and Spicer (2017) suggest that due to insecurities about the outside world, people's attention is increasingly turned inward, and their anxieties also focus on themselves, their performance, their bodies, health, and safety.

The widespread interest in this topic is also evident in the rise of Danish philosopher Svend Brinkmann (2017) as a prominent public intellectual following the release of his book *Stand Firm: Resisting the Self-Improvement Craze*. In this work, he offers a sharp and witty critique of the neoliberal culture of self-actualisation. Brinkmann distils his message into seven points that ironically reference the often clichéd wisdom found in self-help books. He emphasises that rather than focusing on productivity, the pursuit of happiness, or the mantra 'find yourself', we should prioritise finding ways to coexist peacefully with others.

Self-help methods are commonly utilised in clinical practice and are often recommended by professionals to their clients (Gwynne, 2024). However, there is currently no systematic evaluation of their effectiveness, making it challenging to measure their impact. For instance, it is unclear whether reading self-help texts leads to a decrease in the reader's depression or anxiety or improvements in their social relationships or eating habits (Harwood & L'Abate, 2010). Users engage with self-help materials based on simple cause-and-effect principles, focusing on responses. This approach often overlooks environmental and social factors that can influence interpretation and worsen anxiety. Professionals tend to overestimate these negative influences by 'overloading' readers. Finding the right balance is challenging, and creating a definitive model of 'the reader' is impossible.

Self-care activists often reference the American poet and human rights advocate Audre Lorde, who articulated that self-care is a form of self-preservation and a part of political resistance (Lorde, n.d.). While self-care does suggest a focus on the self, it should not be confused with selfishness or hypersensitivity. Recent discussions in scientific literature and popular press have highlighted the contradictions and nuances surrounding the 'selfish' aspects of self-care and self-help concepts (Robson, 2024). For instance, a study involving hundreds of thousands of respondents across 22 European countries argues that altruism, helping others, and volunteering offer several benefits, including improved health, compared to self-focused strategies (de Wit et al., 2022). Lim et al. (2023) examined the 'dark side' of self-care among Asian Generation Z youth. They note this group is heavily influenced by the self-care industry, which often suggests vulnerability. Despite high demand for mental healthcare, professionals are less accessible in Asia than in Western countries, where mental health issues are also taboo. While digital mental health solutions have benefits, online self-care without professional support can lead to problems like death scrolling, binge watching, or gaming. Conversely, some online portals provide information and advice when therapy isn't available (Natividad, 2022). This highlights the challenge of knowing when expert help is necessary and understanding what influences certain therapeutic and self-help perspectives.

'Therapy speak' in popular discourse

In recent decades, there has been a growing call for the demedicalisation of distress as a critical response to the increasing number of mental disorder categories and the expanded use of psychopharmacological agents. This movement advocates for a broader, non-medical approach to mental health which emphasises social factors

(Rose, 2018). This highlights the need for self-help solutions, while there is also a notable trend, especially in the Global North, towards the popularity of therapists, counsellors, life coaches, and other professionals who provide support. As previously discussed, the concepts of the 'wounded self' and the 'celebrated self' define the needs and typical conversations surrounding mental health and well-being services. Western (2012) argues that traditional therapeutic culture is rooted in and contributes to the formation of the 'wounded self'. He references Freud's original perspective, which suggests that therapy aims to transform anxieties and neuroses into what he terms 'ordinary unhappiness' (Freud & Breuer, 1895/2004). However, this also implies that we must live with this 'wound', meaning we must address it and continually work on ourselves and our anxieties. This is the legacy of 'psy-culture', which today also contributes to the need to deal with this wound through the over-psychologisation generated by the internet and social media platforms (Rose, 2018). This is partly supported by the proliferation of psychopathological categories in diagnostic systems and their overuse in public discourse.

On the other hand, the concept of the 'celebrated self', which has emerged from humanistic and positive psychology, spirituality, alternative healing movements, and New Ageism, focuses on positive resources, personal growth, self-actualisation, and self-improvement rather than past traumas (Western, 2012). This idea has become an integral part of therapeutic culture, particularly with the rise of the happiness industry. Furthermore, it is essential to acknowledge that these two types of self, the 'wounded' and the 'celebrated', can coexist within the same discourse, and this phenomenon is becoming increasingly common. This suggests that, on the one hand, the cultural imperative to pursue happiness and self-improvement is always present. On the other hand, there is a discourse that tends to pathologise our experiences, encouraging us to constantly seek out some form of injury, trauma, weakness, or imperfection within ourselves. This creates tension and anxiety that characterise our era and are likely some of the contributors to existential anxiety. In its quest for an object, this anxiety often manifests as health worries.

The increasing visibility of mental health issues in various social arenas is a positive development. However, this awareness alone cannot help everyone and does not necessarily create a sense of safety (de Lange, 2023). The proliferation of psychological and mental health issues in public discourse has led to an increase in health literacy and, therefore, help-seeking and destigmatisation (Fleary et al., 2022). On the other hand, there is also a kind of concept creep, which means that although people's ability to recognise mental health problems has improved, their ability to normalise them, that is, to accept that not all physical and mental changes and subclinical distress are pathological, has deteriorated (Haslam & Tse, 2024). Many social media campaigns, posters, and other public displays tend to be overly simplistic. They often fail to capture the complexities of mental health issues and can focus negatively, encouraging discussions only about the problems. While it is crucial to promote open conversations and encourage individuals to seek help, the lack of available support can lead to significant frustration and anxiety. The growing use of 'therapy speak' in public discourse, alongside messages promoting the pursuit of happiness, conveys a misleading notion that all negative feelings and thoughts should be viewed as indications of some mental disorder or symptom. This perspective fosters an unwarranted sense of vulnerability, which can heighten anxiety and instil a fear of anxiety itself. As a result, individuals may engage in avoidance behaviours, leading to increasingly severe and long-term clinical symptoms and behavioural disorders (Foulkes & Andrews, 2023).

Recent social media discussions on mental health, often called 'psychobabble', have become popular among young people (Nucci, 2025). Terms like 'narcissist', 'gaslighting', 'triggered', 'toxic personality', and 'boundary violation' are increasingly being used. A study analysing the top 25 rap songs from 1998 to 2018 showed mentions of suicide rising from 0% to 25%, depression from 16% to 32%, and mental health metaphors from 8% to 44% (Kresovich et al., 2021). However, many mental health terms are misused publicly (Medaris, 2024). A TikTok survey found that over 80% of videos with #mentalhealth or #mentalhealthtips were misleading, often by unqualified sources that failed to disclose their lack of expertise (Plush Care Content Team, 2024). Over 14% of the content was harmful, encouraging medication use without medical advice. This highlights the need for professionals in online education and innovative solutions to address the challenges of digital culture. Society must also address underlying issues like alienation, loneliness, and lack of meaning, affecting young people and society.

The search for meaning and purpose

According to classical psychodynamic and existentialist approaches, anxiety can make us feel small, insignificant, helpless, abandoned, and threatened by the world (Horney, 1937). One of the leading causes of anxiety is a lack of meaning – the feeling that we cannot find purpose in life (Frankl, 1988). Traditionally, individuals have sought guidance on purpose and meaning from their immediate community and religion. These remain essential resources and significant factors in personal well-being even today (Chamberlain & Zika, 1988b, 1992). As societies become more individualised, there's a growing focus on discovering one's authentic self in secular ways. Early 20th-century psychologists, such as Alfred Adler and Karl Jaspers, viewed 'borderline situations' – times of suffering, pain, and loss – as pivotal moments (Kőváry, 2024). During these times, individuals choose to either succumb to despair or seek a broader, more meaningful perspective. Viktor Frankl (1988) believed that meaning can be found in any circumstance. Over time, this focus on meaning became central to positive psychology and connected to existential psychotherapy.

In recent decades, pursuing a meaningful life has gained significant attention in both therapeutic settings and among the public. Today, more than 30 distinct meaning-centred therapies have been identified in the literature (Vos, 2016). These therapies are primarily grounded in principles of logotherapy; existential analysis;

and various phenomenological, dialogical, and client-centred frameworks. One common criticism of these approaches is that their underlying causes are too complex to validate; they tend to be more philosophical and cannot be linked to a single model (Kővåry, 2024). Many associate a lack of meaning with lower psychological well-being and potential psychopathology, but evidence is often indirect and retrospective, like in cases of trauma or illness. Viktor Frankl's (1988) theory of the 'existential vacuum' highlights a common modern phenomenon – persistent frustration and feelings of emptiness and boredom. While scientific proof is limited, its heuristic value is substantial, supported by the life tragedies of Holocaust survivors, which may explain why many therapies focus on universal values like experience, creativity, and productivity, as Frankl described (Bushkin et al., 2021). While these values are central to the therapeutic goals for many individuals, they have also faced criticism for oversimplifying the complex motivations that influence people's search for meaning (Pytell, 2015). This situation may lead some clients to discontinue therapy as they believe the value dimensions do not resonate with their experiences (Vos, 2016). Consequently, this raises questions for them regarding the very purpose of seeking help. The search for meaning, a fundamental principle and a vital tool, remains valuable in addressing feelings of alienation, insecurity, and anxiety. However, the core values established in the mid-20th century should be revised and supplemented with new values to better align with today's cultural and sociopolitical context.

More recent approaches have addressed meaning and purpose in life, emphasising that effective coping is facilitated when individuals perceive their actions as meaningful, driven by a life purpose, and valuable and important (Scheier et al., 2006). Purpose and meaning may be motivationally interdependent, and some researchers suggest that it is challenging to make an operational distinction between the two constructs, as they are often used interchangeably (Boreham & Schutte, 2023). In any case, since the 1980s, when measurement tools began to be developed, several studies have shown a negative association between purpose and depression in subclinical and clinical samples, even after 10 years of follow-up (Chamberlain & Zika, 1988a; Davison et al., 2012; Ryff, 1989; Wood & Joseph, 2010). Similar results have been found for stress responses, showing that having a purpose in life can have a significant stress-reducing effect (Creswell et al., 2005). A meta-analysis of 89 studies also found that individuals with a diagnosed mental health problem exhibited a stronger negative link between purpose and anxiety, which may worsen their condition by weakening their coping resources (Boreham & Schutte, 2023). Similarly, a connection has been made between a lack of purpose and worse physical health. This implies that having a sense of purpose can lower anxiety and depression and improve overall health behaviours and that a stronger sense of purpose may also decrease avoidance tendencies. In recent years, various initiatives have explored simpler, widely accessible interventions, such as mindfulness techniques, to enhance goal setting and overall happiness. These methods have proven effective in decreasing anxiety and depression (Crego et al., 2021). Additionally, studies have shown that having a clear goal is linked to better health behaviours and a reduction in morbidity and mortality (Kim et al., 2020).

A 4-year study with nearly 13,000 participants found that those with the highest sense of purpose had a 46% lower risk of death, less loneliness and depression, and higher optimism (Kim et al., 2022). However, no links were found between this indicator and other health indicators or behaviours. This indicates that understanding the concepts of purpose and the meaning of life requires further research. Studies emphasise the need for consistent measurement tools, as different questionnaire versions are used, highlighting the necessity for a personalised, comprehensive instrument (Arunjit et al., 2024). This situation presents various challenges, as the interpretation of purpose is deeply rooted in a network of cultural customs and values. Consequently, applying measurement instruments across different cultures and generalising results can be problematic. The same can be said about the spiritual dimension, which is closely linked to purpose and meaning. However, beyond the cultural differences, these issues raise questions about the limitations of psychological theorising, measurement, and the scientific endeavour. Today, these aspects are often challenged and occasionally attacked by esotericism, pop psychology, and, not infrequently, by the internal contradictions within the field of psychological science itself.

The concepts of meaning in life and purpose can be assessed using tools like the Life Engagement Test (Scheier et al., 2006). This test serves as a measurement tool and highlights significant factors such as dispositional optimism, one's social network size, and emotional expression styles. Research has shown that these factors are vital for health behaviours (Non et al., 2020). Furthermore, they may be crucial in managing health anxiety, as they encourage individuals to interact with others, share their feelings, and avoid relying solely on the internet for their often limited and isolated self-monitoring of information (McIntyre et al., 2022). In this way, 'life engagement' can serve as a vital compass for the development of behavioural self-regulation, explicitly adding a proactive dimension of connection with peers, the environment, and the world to the slogans of self-help and self-improvement, as studies conducted during the COVID-19 pandemic have shown.

COVID-19 caused uncertainty and anxiety, offering a chance to reconsider the meaning of life (Aguglia, 2022). A U.S. study conducted early in the pandemic found that social media use protected against social isolation, with a stronger sense of purpose in life being linked to less isolation (Helm et al., 2022). While social media reduced social loneliness, it has not alleviated emotional loneliness; increased usage sometimes heightens personal disconnection, thereby raising emotional loneliness (Bonsaksen et al., 2021). However, active use helped people feel less alone, strengthening social bonds. Research on youth during the pandemic confirms that searching for the meaning of life can be both natural and potentially harmful, depending on motivation (Karayigit, 2024; Reker, 2000). Curiosity and openness usually enhance well-being, while depression and rumination tend to diminish it. Older adults often report a stronger sense of purpose, but their search for meaning sometimes correlates with lower well-being, possibly due to shorter life expectancy. A 'crisis of meaning' involves feelings of emptiness and lack of purpose (Reker & Chamberlain, 2000; Schnell, 2009). When social media is used to seek reassurance, it should promote positive goals and healthy behaviours rather than risk or addiction. Focusing on positive meaning can help reduce anxiety and depression (Schnell & Krampe, 2022).

Fostering connectedness and resonance

In recent decades, positive psychology has encountered several criticisms and has been constructively integrated into more contemporary approaches (Wong, 2011; van Zyl et al., 2023). The third wave of positive psychology aims to move beyond an individualistic perspective by considering the systems and environments that influence and define the individual. This approach emphasises a more interdisciplinary and methodologically diverse perspective (Lomas et al., 2021). This includes the theory of Steger (2024), who, after the first 25 years of positive psychology, heralded a new era of 'Regenerative Positive Psychology'. Their starting point was that, over the last quarter of a century, life satisfaction has increased, and indicators of happiness have improved. Similarly, depression and suicide rates have declined worldwide. However, indicators of anxiety have increased, as has alcohol consumption. This contradictory picture also highlights the uncertainty of measurement tools and the question of the validity of 'big data' surveys on a global scale. Steger (2024) cites as a further problem the criticism by many that 80% of positive psychology studies focus on the individual, as if the isolated individual were the primary actor and do not consider, for example, global indicators of happiness, while environmental conditions such as pollution or global warming have deteriorated significantly. The author highlights that individual-centredness is prominent in the field, exemplified by the 50 most-cited articles in the *Journal of Positive Psychology*, where 96% focus solely on the individual. This heavy emphasis on the individual can lead to feelings of guilt and anxiety, as discussed in various sections of our volume. Regenerative positive psychology seeks to identify the resources essential for maintaining health and well-being not just at the individual level but also at the societal, community, and even planetary levels. The core idea is prioritising their sustainability instead of depleting these resources to pursue growth and productivity.

Another new concept in the third wave of positive psychology is Maurer's (2024) Organismic Systems Theory (OST). This theory provides a holistic framework that utilises a multi-level and broad approach to connectedness. It combines a systems approach with organismic theory, drawing from biology, psychology, and the philosophy of science. The key principles of OST include individual activity, functionality, integration, emergence, dynamism, self-regulation, interconnectedness, holism, boundaries, subjectivity, and adaptation. This meta-theory effectively addresses the often-criticised individualistic focus of positive psychology by elevating the discussion to a systems level. It also provides a valuable framework for understanding health anxiety and the safety-seeking behaviours explored in this volume. By highlighting the connection with the environment, the theory suggests that individuals are responsible for their health and the health of their surroundings without feeling abandoned or disconnected. Instead, they are viewed as organismic beings and active agents.

One of the challenges we face today is accepting that, despite the remarkable technological advances of recent decades, we cannot fully control the world around us. We are still confronted with many unpredictable and unexpected events. Acknowledging and accepting life's inherent uncertainty are crucial in reducing anxiety and fostering a sense of internal safety. According to contemporary German sociologist Hartmut Rosa (2019, 2020), the concept of *resonance* can help address various crises. Resonance refers to the ability to engage with the world without trying to control it, turning away from it, or isolating ourselves from it. Rosa's critical sociological theory, influenced by the Frankfurt School of sociology and critical philosophy (including thinkers such as Adorno, Fromm, Marcuse, Habermas, and Honneth), argues that capitalist modernity has caused crises at the political, environmental, and interpersonal levels. In this context, fostering a state of resonance can play a significant role in addressing these challenges. Rosa examines the relationship between personal experience and acceleration dynamics, which he discussed in his earlier work (Rosa, 2013). He proposes that the desire to connect with others is an inherent human drive. However, he also notes that when this desire becomes unregulated or excessive, it can lead to hostility, violence, and aggressive authoritarian behaviour. Nevertheless, the theory does not fully explain the mechanisms behind this phenomenon nor clarify whether the often-criticised functions of capitalist development and acceleration can be replaced by resonance. Additionally, it remains uncertain whether resonance has the emancipatory potential necessary for meaningful transformation (Anderson, 2023).

Rosa (2018) begins with the concept of alienation, which describes a connection to the world that lacks responsiveness and meaning. In a state of alienation, the relationship between the self and the world can feel indifferent or even hostile, leading to issues such as depression or burnout. Rosa emphasises that improving these negative emotions and attitudes relies on acknowledging that there is always an affective dimension to our connection with the world – a resonance indicating that we are impacted by external factors – and an emotional dimension representing our response to those influences. In addition to the psychological, cognitive, and social aspects, resonance also has a bodily dimension. The meaningful, reciprocal relationship between the self and the world is significant in transformation and identity formation. This could explain why people often say that personal relationships, artistic experiences, or other important events have profoundly changed their lives. A key characteristic of these experiences is that they occur partly outside conscious control and cannot always be predicted. Therefore, to be genuinely moved by the world around us and foster positive resonance, we must be open and ready to engage with and receive these experiences.

Today, many people withdraw from interactions with others because they perceive the world as a frightening and dangerous place. This sense of alienation intensifies feelings of emptiness inside the individual, which can increase anxiety and lead to various psychosomatic symptoms. In this detached state, the lack of genuine attachment worsens the fear of losing connection to oneself. This fear can manifest as health anxiety, worsening symptoms, or the development of addictions and self-harm (Mushtaq et al., 2014).

A crucial tool for reducing anxiety and promoting a sense of safety is the development of meaningful relationships. According to Rosa (2018), the starting point for connection and achieving a state of resonance is not a place of complete harmony or 'perfect happiness', as this does not provide sufficient motivation to connect. Instead, it begins with a deficit that encompasses the need for personal development and openness to differences. Only then can positive, mutual transformation and adaptation occur. However, this initial state must reflect only a moderate lack, with needs expressed in a positive manner. A strong sense of dissonance and conflict can be off-putting and hinder the ability to attune to one another, creating the desired resonance.

The first step to finding safety and reducing anxiety is to dissolve isolating, defensive attitudes and to become open to being 'touched' by others (Rosa, 2018). This openness fosters the development of mutually beneficial relationships and a deeper resonance with the environment (Höffken, 2024). By doing so, individuals can prevent a state of isolation, which many wrongly perceive as a means of seeking safety as a defence against the world's dangers. However, in the long run, isolation results in an emptiness within the self. This empty self, lacking stable content, becomes fragile and vulnerable. Without substance, it often fills itself arbitrarily with surrounding cultural influences, frequently adopting meaningless content foreign to the self which may undermine its stability and well-being (Cushman, 1990).

In our world, genuine resonance is likely what draws the most people. However, the challenge is to determine how far and effectively social and political frameworks can support this resonance beyond the individual psychological level. This issue reflects the dilemmas faced by humanistic, existential, and positive psychology, all of which have been scrutinised concerning their evidence-based foundations versus idealistic aspirations. Nevertheless, Rosa's theory of resonance is particularly relevant today, emphasising our relationship with the world. It addresses the environmental crisis, a significant source of anxiety and concern related to the deterioration of our connection with the world and, by extension, ourselves. It is also crucial to consider balancing the need for connection and resonance and preventing its excesses. Without proper balance, this need can manifest in dangerous, exclusionary, and nationalistic movements (Anderson, 2023).

Genuine connection and resonance are vital for fostering and valuing authenticity (Plesa, 2023). Nevertheless, there is no straightforward formula or instant solution; it is undoubtedly not about exerting control at all costs. The intense desire for control that many people seek today may not be beneficial. As we attempt to control the world more, everything becomes more predictable, resulting in fewer unexpected and novel events. These events capture our interest, motivate and inspire us, and ultimately help us evolve. This idea is also reflected in the recent theory of *psychological richness*, which expands beyond the concepts of happiness and meaningfulness (Oishi & Westgate, 2022). It suggests that engaging in experiences that change one's perspective contributes to a psychologically meaningful life. The authors argue that psychological richness is crucial to achieving a fulfilling life, alongside both hedonic and eudaimonic well-being. Psychological richness is characterised by curiosity, holistic thinking, and a liberal outlook. A metaphor attributed to Kierkegaard suggests that the door to happiness opens outward towards the world and connection (Kierkegaard, 1843/1959). To experience psychological richness and resonance, the world must be accessible, tangible, and experienceable. This accessibility is possible only through mutual relationships that we must actively and continually cultivate. Such relationships can give us a sense of balanced control, effectively managing our anxieties about our bodies and health and ultimately leading to a sense of inner peace and safety.

Conclusion

People often encounter difficulties in finding purpose and a sense of safety today, as many see the world as a complex and unpredictable place. However, the previous focus of psychology on individual meaning-making and well-being often overlooked the influence of social, economic, and political systems. A broader perspective on well-being should consider how systemic inequalities affect people's ability to find purpose and flourish. The differences among contemporary therapeutic approaches relate to the notions of the 'wounded' and 'celebrated' self. The rise of 'psy-culture' – encompassing pop psychology, self-help books, lifestyle therapies, and 'happiness training' – can enhance health literacy and empowerment; however, it may also lead to new health issues by overlooking negative emotions, promoting inauthenticity, and eroding resilience. Critics argue that the neoliberal view of happiness shifts attention from power structures to self-management, encouraging individuals to focus on personal well-being rather than critically examining social relationships. Society's suffering becomes privatised and psychologised instead of being addressed as a societal issue. This tendency isolates individuals, depoliticises society, and erodes solidarity, causing everyone to see their happiness as a personal matter. The third wave of positive psychology explores these matters from multiple perspectives, aiming for a comprehensive, multidisciplinary approach to well-being that tackles methodological and contextual challenges. Unlike many traditional approaches that concentrate solely on individuals, a promising new wave of theories highlights resonance and connectedness as adaptive strategies to reduce health anxiety and foster safety.

REFERENCES

Abramowitz, J. S., & Braddock, A. E. (2011). *Hypochondriasis and health anxiety*. Hogrefe Publishing.

Ackerley, B. (2024, April 3). Anxiety really has increased over the past 10 years – but why? *New Scientist*. https://www.newscientist.com/article/mg26234851–900-anxiety-really-has-increased-over-the-past-10-years-but-why/

Adams, K. G. (1935). *Don't be afraid*. Covici-Friede.

Agence France-Presse. (2021, August 25). Xiaoice is the AI chatbot that millions of lonely Chinese are turning to for comfort. *Firstpost*. https://www.firstpost.com/tech/news-analysis/xiaoice-is-the-ai-chatbot-that-millions-of-lonely-chinese-are-turning-to-for-comfort–9910921.html

Aguglia, E. (2022). Reshaping our meaning in life to cope with uncertainty. *Journal of Psychopathology*, *28*(1–2).

Ahadzadeh, A. S., Rafik-Galea, S., Alavi, M., & Amini, M. (2018). Relationship between body mass index, body image, and fear of negative evaluation: Moderating role of self-esteem. *Health Psychology Open*, *5*(1), 2055102918774251. https://doi.org/10.1177/2055102918774251

Ahmed, A., Hassan, A., Aziz, S., Abd-Alrazaq, A. A., Ali, N., Alzubaidi, M., Al-Thani, D., Elhusein, B., Siddig, M. A., Ahmed, M., & Househ, M. (2023). Chatbot features for anxiety and depression: A scoping review. *Health Informatics Journal*, *29*(1), 14604582221146719. https://doi.org/10.1177/14604582221146719

Ajana, B. (2020). Personal metrics: Users' experiences and perceptions of self-tracking practices and data. *Social Science Information*, *59*(4), 654–678. https://doi.org/10.1177/0539018420959522

Akbari, H., Mohammadi, M., & Hosseini, A. (2023). Disease-related stigma, stigmatizers, causes, and consequences: A systematic review. *Iranian Journal of Public Health*, *52*(10), 2042–2054. https://doi.org/10.18502/ijph.v52i10.13842

Akerlof, K., DeBono, R., Berry, P., Leiserowitz, A., Roser-Renouf, C., Clarke, K.-L., Rogaeva, A., Nisbet, M. C., Weathers, M. R., & Maibach, E. W. (2010). Public perceptions of climate change as a human health risk: Surveys of the United States, Canada, and Malta. *International Journal of Environmental Research and Public Health*, *7*(7), 2559–2606. https://doi.org/10.3390/ijerph7062559

Akgül, G., & Ergin, D. A. (2020). Adolescents' and parents' anxiety during COVID-19: Is there a role of cyberchondriasis and emotion regulation through the internet? *Current Psychology*. https://doi.org/10.1007/s12144-020-01229-7

Alaszewski, A. (2005). Risk communication: Identifying the importance of social context. *Health, Risk and Society*, *7*(2), 101–105. https://doi.org/10.1080/13698570500148905

Alberga, A. S., Nutter, S., MacInnis, C., Ellard, J. H., & Russell-Mayhew, S. (2019). Examining weight bias among practicing Canadian family physicians. *Obesity Facts*, *12*(6), 632–638. https://doi.org/10.1159/000503751

Albert, S. L., Massar, R. E., Cassidy, O., Fennelly, K., Jay, M., Massey, P. M., & Bragg, M. A. (2024). Body positivity, physical health, and emotional well-being discourse on social media: Content analysis of Lizzo's Instagram. *JMIR Formative Research*, *8*, e60541. https://doi.org/10.2196/60541

Albrecht, G. A. (2011). Chronic environmental change: Emerging 'psychoterratic' syndromes. In I. Weissbecker (Ed.), *Climate change and human well-being* (pp. 43–56). Springer New York.

Albrecht, G. A. (2019). *Earth emotions: New words for a new world*. Cornell University Press.

Allen, W. (2013, January 12). Hypochondria: An inside look. *The New York Times*. https://www.nytimes.com/2013/01/13/opinion/sunday/hypochondria-an-inside-look.html?_r=0

Alleva, J. M., & Tylka, T. L. (2021). Body functionality: A review of the literature. *Body Image*, *36*, 149–171. https://doi.org/10.1016/j.bodyim.2020.11.006

Alowais, S. A., Alghamdi, S. S., Alsuhebany, N., Alqathani, T., Alshaya, A. I., Almohareb, S. N., Aldairem, A., Alrashed, M., Saleh, K. B., Badreldin, H. A., Al Yami, M. S., Al Harbi, S., & Albekairy, A. M. (2023). Revolutionizing healthcare: The role of artificial intelligence in clinical practice. *BMC Medical Education, 23*, 689. https://doi.org/10.1186/s12909-023-04698-z

Ambwani, S., Shippe, M., Gao, Z., & Austin, S. B. (2019). Is #cleaneating a healthy or harmful dietary strategy? Perceptions of clean eating and associations with disordered eating among young adults. *Journal of Eating Disorders, 7*, 17. https://doi.org/10.1186/s40337-019-0246-2

American Psychiatric Association. (2013). *Diagnostic and statistical manual of mental disorders* (5th ed.). https://doi.org/10.1176/appi.books.9780890425596

Amos, C., Pentina, I., Hawkins, T. G., & Davis, N. (2014). "Natural" labeling and consumers' sentimental pastoral notion. *Journal of Product & Brand Management*, *23*(4/5), 268–281. https://doi.org/10.1108/JPBM-03-2014-0516

Andersen, T. O., Langstrup, H., & Lomborg, S. (2020). Experiences with wearable activity data during self-care by chronic heart patients: Qualitative study. *Journal of Medical Internet Research*, *22*(7), e15873. https://doi.org/10.2196/15873

Anderson, A. (2023). The moral and political challenges of Hartmut Rosa's theory of resonance. *The Journal of Chinese Sociology*, *10*(6). https://doi.org/10.1186/s40711-023-00182-9

ANSA. (2020, March 5). Coronavirus: CNN contagion map distorts reality – Di Maio. *ANSA*. https://www.ansa.it/english/news/2020/03/05/coronaviruscnn-contagion-map-distorts-reality-di-maio_c037fd04–58c7–467d-8019–6ba99e7f79fd.html

Arnot, G., Pitt, H., McCarthy, S., Warner, E., & Thomas, S. (2024). "You can't really separate these risks, our environment, our animals and us": Australian children's perceptions of the risks of the climate crisis. *Health Promotion International*, *39*(2), daae023. https://doi.org/10.1093/heapro/daae023

Arunjit, S., Balthip, K., & Latour, J. M. (2024). Measuring the purpose in life in the adult population: A scoping review. *Belitung Nursing Journal*, *10*(2), 126–133. https://doi.org/10.33546/bnj.3176

Arya, B., & Kumar, H. (2023). An investigation of climate change, eco-anxiety, and risk perception in the context of the theory of planned behaviour. *IOP Conference Series:*

Earth and Environmental Science, 1279(1), 012020. https://doi.org/10.1088/1755-1315/1279/1/012020

Atillah, I. E. (2023, March 31). Man ends his life after an AI chatbot 'encouraged' him to sacrifice himself to stop climate change. *EuroNews*. https://www.euronews.com/next/2023/03/31/man-ends-his-life-after-an-ai-chatbot-encouraged-him-to-sacrifice-himself-to-stop-climate-

Auden, W. H. (1947). *The age of anxiety: A baroque eclogue*. Random House.

Avalos, L., Tylka, T. L., & Wood-Barcalow, N. (2005). The body appreciation scale: Development and psychometric evaluation. *Body Image*, *2*(3), 285–297. https://doi.org/10.1016/j.bodyim.2005.06.002

Babic, A., de Valck, K., & Lowrey, T. M. (2014). Against the grain: A study of social identity reconstruction in online 'gluten-free living' communities. *Presented at the Association for Consumer Research Conference, Baltimore, USA*, October 2014. https://doi.org/10.13140/RG.2.1.2233.3284.

Bachl, M., Link, E., Mangold, F., & Stier, S. (2024). Search engine use for health-related purposes: Behavioral data on online health information-seeking in Germany. *Health Communication*. https://doi.org/10.1080/10410236.2024.2309810

Bacon, L. (2010). *Health at every size: The surprising truth about your weight*. BenBella Books.

Bagayogo, I. P., Interian, A., & Escobar, J. I. (2013). Transcultural aspects of somatic symptoms in the context of depressive disorders. In R. D. Alarcón (Ed.), *Cultural psychiatry, Vol. 33: Advances in psychosomatic medicine* (pp. 64–74). Karger.

Bailey, R. (2024). Why health anxiety needs NICE clinical guidelines. *The Lancet Psychiatry*, *11*(3), 164–165. https://doi.org/10.1016/S2215-0366(23)00404–2

Bajcar, B., & Babiak, J. (2021). Self-esteem and cyberchondria: The mediation effects of health anxiety and obsessive–compulsive symptoms in a community sample. *Current Psychology*, *40*(11), 2820–2831. https://doi.org/10.1007/s12144-019-00216-x

Baldemor, R. V. V., Ong, A. K. S., German, J. D., Bautista, N. S., Alonso, M. L. V., & Alidio, O. J. P. (2024). Health belief and behavioral analysis of fad diets: A perspective from younger generations in a developing country. *Foods*, *13*(12), 1858. https://doi.org/10.3390/foods13121858

Bandelow, B. (2017). Comparison of the DSM-5 and ICD-10: Panic and other anxiety disorders. *CNS Spectrums*, *22*(5), 404–406. https://doi.org/10.1017/S1092852917000116

Barbek, R., Henning, S., Ludwig, J., & von dem Knesebeck, O. (2022b). Ethnic and migration-related inequalities in health anxiety: A systematic review and meta-analysis. *Frontiers in Psychology*, *13*, 960256. https://doi.org/10.3389/fpsyg.2022.960256

Barbek, R. M. E., Makowski, A. C., & von dem Knesebeck, O. (2022a). Social inequalities in health anxiety: A systematic review and meta-analysis. *Journal of Psychosomatic Research*, *153*, 110706. https://doi.org/10.1016/j.jpsychores.2021.110706

Barskova, T., & Oesterreich, R. (2009). Post-traumatic growth in people living with a serious medical condition and its relations to physical and mental health: A systematic review. *Disability and Rehabilitation*, *31*(21), 1709–1733. https://doi.org/10.1080/09638280902738441

Barthes, R. (2000). *Camera lucida: Reflections on photography*. Vintage.

Bauman, Z. (1998). *Globalization: The human consequences*. Columbia University Press.

Bauman, Z. (2006). *Liquid times: Living in the age of uncertainty*. Polity Press.

Bauman, Z. (2017). *Retrotopia*. Polity Press.

Baur, S. (1989). *Hypochondria: Woeful imaginings*. University of California Press.

Baxter, A. J., Scott, K. M., Ferrari, A. J., Norman, R. E., Vos, T., & Whiteford, H. A. (2014). Challenging the myth of an "epidemic" of common mental disorders: Trends in the global prevalence of anxiety and depression between 1990 and 2010. *Depression and Anxiety*, *31*(6), 506–516. https://doi.org/10.1002/da.22230

Bayram, M. H., Barcin-Guzeldere, K. H., EdeCintesun, E., & Margot-Celik, Z. (2024). Exploring the interplay between social media addiction, mindful eating, intuitive eating, orthorexia nervosa, and mental health in young adults. *The North African Journal of Food and Nutrition Research, 8*(18), 70–79. https://doi.org/10.51745/najfnr.8.18.70–79

Beard, G. M. (1881). *American nervousness: Its causes and consequences, a supplement to nervous exhaustion (neurasthenia)*. Putnam.

Beck, U. (1992). *Risk society: Towards a new modernity*. Sage.

Beck, U., Giddens, A., & Lash, S. (1994). *Reflexive modernization: Politics, tradition and aesthetics in the modern social order*. Polity Press.

Beeker, T., Mills, C., Bhugra, D., Te Meerman, S., Thoma, S., Heinze, M., & Von Peter, S. (2021). Psychiatrization of society: A conceptual framework and call for transdisciplinary research. *Frontiers in Psychiatry, 12*, 645556. https://doi.org/10.3389/fpsyt.2021.645556

Bell, R. A., Kravitz, R. L., Thom, D. H., & Azari, R. (2002). Unmet expectations for care and the patient–physician relationship. *Journal of General Internal Medicine, 17*(11), 817–824. https://doi.org/10.1046/j.1525-1497.2002.10319.x

Belling, C. (2006). Hypochondriac hermeneutics: Medicine and the anxiety of interpretation. *Literature and Medicine, 25*(2), 376–401. https://doi.org/10.1353/lm.2007.0000

Belling, C. F. (2012). *A condition of doubt: The meanings of hypochondria*. Oxford University Press.

Bendell, J., & Read, R. (Eds.). (2021). *Deep adaptation*. Polity Press.

BenendenHealth. (2023). *Should you Google your symptoms?* https://www.benenden.co.uk/be-healthy/body/dr-google-will-see-you-now/

Benke, C., Wallenfels, L. M., Bleichhardt, G. M., & Melzig, C. A. (2024). Health anxiety amplifies fearful responses to illness-related imagery. *Scientific Reports, 14*(1), 4345. https://doi.org/10.1038/s41598-024-54985-y

Bennett, K. K., Compas, B. E., Beckjord, E., & Glinder, J. G. (2005). Self-blame and distress among women with newly diagnosed breast cancer. *Journal of Behavioral Medicine, 28*(4), 313–323. https://doi.org/10.1007/s10865-005-9000-0

Bensing, J. M., & Verhaak, P. F. M. (2006). Somatisation: A joint responsibility of doctor and patient. *The Lancet, 367*(9509), 452–454. https://doi.org/10.1016/S0140-6736(06)68155–5

Berge, L. I., Skogen, J. C., Sulo, G., Igland, J., Wilhelmsen, I., Vollset, S. E., Tell, G. S., & Knudsen, A. K. (2016). Health anxiety and risk of ischaemic heart disease: A prospective cohort study linking the Hordaland Health Study (HUSK) with the Cardiovascular Diseases in Norway (CVDNOR) project. *BMJ Open, 6*(11), e012914. https://doi.org/10.1136/bmjopen-2016-012914

Berger, B. E., Kapella, M. C., & Larson, J. L. (2011). The experience of stigma in chronic obstructive pulmonary disease. *Western Journal of Nursing Research, 33*(7), 916–932. https://doi.org/10.1177/0193945910384602

Bericat, E. (2016). The sociology of emotions: Four decades of progress. *Current Sociology, 64*(3), 491–513. https://doi.org/10.1177/0011392115588355

Berlin, S. (2022, October 27). Disney's newest film *Reflect* stirs debate online about plus-size lead. *Newsweek*. https://www.newsweek.com/disney-newest-film-reflect-stirs-debate-online-plus-size-lead-1755186

Berry, D. C. (2004). *Risk, communication and health psychology*. Open University Press.

Blanding, M. (2019, February 6). The strange case of Dr. Ho Man Kwok. *Colgate Magazine*. https://news.colgate.edu/magazine/2019/02/06/the-strange-case-of-dr-ho-man-kwok/

Blum, B. (2020, January 29). When did self-help books become literary? Beth Blum on a debate over bookish advice that goes as far back as the Renaissance. *Literary Hub*. https://lithub.com/when-did-self-help-books-become-literary/

Boero, N. (2012). *Killer fat: Media, medicine, and morals in the American 'Obesity Epidemic'*. Rutgers University Press.

Boldi, A., & Rapp, A. (2022). Quantifying the body: Body image, body awareness and self-tracking technologies. In K. Wac & S. Wulfovich (Eds.), *Quantifying quality of life (health informatics)*. Springer. https://doi.org/10.1007/978-3-030-94212-0_9

Boluda-Verdú, I., Senent-Valero, M., Casas-Escolano, M., Matijasevich, A., & Pastor-Valero, M. (2022). Fear for the future: Eco-anxiety and health implications, a systematic review. *Journal of Environmental Psychology*, *84*, 101904. https://doi.org/10.1016/j.jenvp.2022.101904

Bonanno, G. A. (2004). Loss, trauma, and human resilience: Have we underestimated the human capacity to thrive after extremely aversive events? *American Psychologist*, *59*(1), 20–28. https://doi.org/10.1037/0003-066X.59.1.20

Bond, R. R., Mulvenna, M. D., Potts, C., O'Neill, S., Ennis, E., & Torous, J. (2023). Digital transformation of mental health services. *npj Mental Health Research*, *2*, 13. https://doi.org/10.1038/s44184-023-00033-y

Bonsaksen, T., Ruffolo, M., Leung, J., Price, D., Thygesen, H., Schoultz, M., & Geirdal, A. Ø. (2021). Loneliness and its association with social media use during the COVID-19 outbreak. *Social Media + Society*, *7*(3). https://doi.org/10.1177/20563051211033821

Bordo, S. (2004). *Unbearable weight: Feminism, Western culture, and the body*. University of California Press.

Boreham, I. D., & Schutte, N. S. (2023). The relationship between purpose in life and depression and anxiety: A meta-analysis. *Journal of Clinical Psychology*, *79*(12), 2736–2767. https://doi.org/10.1002/jclp.23576

Bourke, J. (2005). *Fear: A cultural history*. Virago.

Bracke, S. (2016). Bouncing back: Vulnerability and resistance in times of resilience. In J. Butler, Z. Gambetti, & L. Sabsay (Eds.), *Vulnerability in resistance* (pp. 52–75). Duke University Press.

Brady, R. E., & Braz, A. N. (2023). Challenging interactions between patients with severe health anxiety and the healthcare system: A qualitative investigation. *Journal of Primary Care & Community Health*, *14*, 21501319231214876.

Bratland, K. M., Wien, C., & Sandanger, T. M. (2024). Exploring online health information seeking behaviour (OHISB) among young adults: A scoping review protocol. *BMJ Open*, *14*, e074894. https://doi.org/10.1136/bmjopen-2023-074894

Bratman, S. (1997, September/October). Health food junkie. *Yoga Journal*, 42–50.

Brewster, M. L., & Sklar, M. (2022). Brand, community, lifestyle: Fashioning an authentic, body-positive influencer brand on Instagram. *Fashion, Style & Popular Culture*, *9*(4), 501–521. https://doi.org/10.1386/fspc_00158_1

Breznitz, S. (1983). The seven kinds of denial. In S. Breznitz (Ed.), *The denial of stress* (pp. 257–280). International Universities Press.

Brickhouse, T. C., & Smith, N. D. (1994). *Plato's Socrates*. Oxford University Press. https://doi.org/10.1093/0195101113.001.0001

Brinkmann, S. (2017). *Stand firm: Resisting the self-improvement craze*. Polity Press.

Brookes, G., & Baker, P. (2021). *Obesity in the news: Language and representation in the press*. Cambridge University Press.

Brown, R. C. H., & Savulescu, J. (2019). Responsibility in healthcare across time and agents. *Journal of Medical Ethics*, *45*(10), 636–644. https://doi.org/10.1136/medethics-2019-105382

Brown, R. J., Skelly, N., & Chew-Graham, C. A. (2019). Online health research and health anxiety: A systematic review and conceptual integration. *Clinical Psychology: Science and Practice*. https://doi.org/10.1111/cpsp.12299

Brunier, A., & Drysdale, C. (2022, March 2). COVID-19 pandemic triggers 25% increase in prevalence of anxiety and depression worldwide. *World Health Organization*. https://www.who.int/news/item/02-03-2022-covid-19-pandemic-triggers-25-increase-in-prevalence-of-anxiety-and-depression-worldwide

Brzozowski, A., & Crossey, B. P. (2024). Maladaptive emotion regulation strategies mediate the relationship between biased cognitions and depression. *Journal of Behavioral and Cognitive Therapy*, *34*(1), 100485. https://doi.org/10.1016/j.jbct.2024.100485

Burychka, D., Miragall, M., & Baños, R. M. (2021). Towards a comprehensive understanding of body image: Integrating positive body image, embodiment, and self-compassion. *Psychologica Belgica*, *61*(1), 248–261. https://doi.org/10.5334/pb.1057

Bushkin, H., van Niekerk, R., & Stroud, L. (2021). Searching for meaning in chaos: Viktor Frankl's story. *European Journal of Psychology*, *17*(3), 233–242. https://doi.org/10.5964/ejop.5439

Butler, J. (1993). *Bodies that matter*. Routledge.

Byniarski, A., & Brock, S. (2022, October 29). How anti-fatness crept into the environmental sustainability movement. *The Guardian*. https://www.theguardian.com/environment/2022/oct/29/fat-people-metabolic-food-waste

Callebaut, L., Molyneux, P., & Alexander, T. (2016). The relationship between self-blame for the onset of a chronic physical health condition and emotional distress: A systematic literature review. *Clinical Psychology & Psychotherapy*, *24*(4), 965–986. https://doi.org/10.1002/cpp.2061

Cambardella, C., Fath, B. D., Werdenigg, A., Gulas, C., & Katzmair, H. (2020). Assessing the operationalization of cultural theory through surveys investigating the social aspects of climate change policy making. *Weather, Climate, and Society*, *12*(4), 651–665. https://doi.org/10.1175/WCAS-D-19-0103.1

Campbell, T., & Sitze, A. (Eds.). (2013). *Biopolitics: A reader*. Duke University Press.

Cárdenas-Torres, F. I., Cabrera-Chávez, F., Figueroa-Salcido, O. G., & Ontiveros, N. (2021). Non-celiac gluten sensitivity: An update. *Medicina (Kaunas)*, *57*(6), 526. https://doi.org/10.3390/medicina57060526

Carey, T. A. (2020, December 18). Why are self-help books not so helpful after all? It's all about the self. *Psychology Today*. https://www.psychologytoday.com/intl/blog/in-control/202012/why-are-self-help-books-not-so-helpful-after-all

Carlisle, S., Henderson, G., & Hanlon, P. W. (2009). 'Wellbeing': A collateral casualty of modernity? *Social Science and Medicine*, *69*(10), 1556–1560. https://doi.org/10.1016/j.socscimed.2009.08.029

Cash, T. F. (2004). Body image: Past, present, and future. *Body Image*, *1*(1), 1–5. https://doi.org/10.1016/S1740-1445(03)00011–1

Casson, N., Cameron, L., Mauro, I., Friesen-Hughes, K., & Rocque, R. (2023). Perceptions of the health impacts of climate change among Canadians. *BMC Public Health*, *23*(1), 212. https://doi.org/10.1186/s12889-023-15105-z

Castellini, G., & Graffigna, G. (2022). Evolution of milk consumption and its psychological determinants: A mini-review. *Frontiers in Nutrition*, *9*, 845154. https://doi.org/10.3389/fnut.2022.845154

Castillo, S. M., & Santa-Cruz-Espinoza, H. (2024). Stigma and mental health in patients with a cancer diagnosis. *Enfermeria Global*, *73*. https://doi.org/10.6018/eglobal.563831

Cederström, C., & Spicer, A. (2015). *The wellness syndrome*. Polity Press.

Cederström, C., & Spicer, A. (2017). *Desperately seeking self-improvement: A year inside the optimization movement*. OR Books.

Chamberlain, K. (2004). Food and health: Expanding the agenda for health psychology. *Journal of Health Psychology*, *9*(4), 467–481. https://doi.org/10.1177/1359105304044030

Chamberlain, K., & Lyons, A. (Eds.). (2022). *Routledge international handbook of critical issues in health and illness*. Routledge.

Chamberlain, K., & Zika, S. (1988a). Measuring meaning in life: An examination of three scales. *Personality and Individual Differences*, *9*(3), 589–596. https://doi.org/10.1016/0191-8869(88)90157–2

Chamberlain, K., & Zika, S. (1988b). Religiosity, life meaning and wellbeing: Some relationships in a sample of women. *Journal for the Scientific Study of Religion*, *27*(3), 411–420. https://doi.org/10.2307/1387379

Chamberlain, K., & Zika, S. (1992). Religiosity, meaning in life, and psychological well-being. In J. F. Schumaker (Ed.), *Religion and mental health* (pp. 138–148). Oxford University Press.

Chambers, L. A., Rueda, S., Baker, D. N., Wilson, M. G., Deutsch, R., Raeifar, E., Rourke, S. B., & Team, T. S. R. (2015). Stigma, HIV and health: A qualitative synthesis. *BMC Public Health, 15*, 848. https://doi.org/10.1186/s12889-015-2197-0
Chandler, D., & Reid, J. (2016). *The neoliberal subject: Resilience, adaptation and vulnerability*. Rowman & Littlefield.
Chapman, B. P., Fiscella, K., Kawachi, I., Duberstein, P., & Muennig, P. (2013). Emotion suppression and mortality risk over a 12-year follow-up. *Journal of Psychosomatic Research, 75*(4), 381–385. https://doi.org/10.1016/j.jpsychores.2013.07.014
Chén, O. Y., & Roberts, B. (2021). Personalized health care and public health in the digital age. *Frontiers in Digital Health, 3*, 595704. https://doi.org/10.3389/fdgth.2021.595704
Chen, S. (2024, August 29). New campaign aims to address racist stereotypes around MSG. *Axios San Francisco*. https://www.axios.com/local/san-francisco/2024/08/29/chinatown-msg-chinese-restaurant-syndrome-nejm
Cheng, C. T., Ho, S. M., Hou, Y. C., Lai, Y., & Wang, G. L. (2020). Constructive, illusory, and distressed posttraumatic growth among survivors of breast cancer: A 7-year growth trajectory study. *Journal of Health Psychology, 25*(13–14), 2233–2243. https://doi.org/10.1177/1359105318793199
Cheng, M. S. (2007). Undoing common ground: Argumentation in self-help books. *OSSA Conference Archive, 25*. https://scholar.uwindsor.ca/ossaarchive/OSSA7/papersandcommentaries/25
Cheston, K. B. A. (2022). (Dis)respect and shame in the context of 'medically unexplained' illness. *Journal of Evaluation in Clinical Practice, 28*(5), 909–916. https://doi.org/10.1111/jep.13740
Chesworth, B. (2022, May 2). Health anxiety and the intolerance of uncertainty: How the fear of the unknown is making you more anxious about your health. *Psychology Today*. https://www.psychologytoday.com/us/blog/managing-health-anxiety/202205/health-anxiety-and-the-intolerance-uncertainty
Cheung, C. C., & Saad, M. (2024). Wearable devices and psychological wellbeing – are we overthinking it? *Journal of the American Heart Association, 13*(15), e035962. https://doi.org/10.1161/JAHA.124.035962
China Daily Global. (2020, January 25). 'Chinese restaurant syndrome' generating a different reaction. *China Daily Global*. https://global.chinadaily.com.cn/a/202001/25/WS5e2b71c6a310128217273284.html
Chiodo, S. (2022). Quantified self as epistemological anarchism. *Philosophia, 50*(2), 1–21. https://doi.org/10.1007/s11406-022-00483-2
Cho, S. E., Kwon, M., & Kim, S. (2022). Influence of diabetes knowledge, self-stigma, and self-care behavior on quality of life in patients with diabetes. *Healthcare, 10*, 1983–1992. https://doi.org/10.3390/healthcare10101983
Choe, E. K., Lee, N. B., Lee, B., & Kientz, J. A. (2014). Understanding quantified-selfers' practices in collecting and exploring personal data. In *Proceedings of the 32nd annual ACM conference on human factors in computing systems* (pp. 1143–1152). ACM. https://doi.org/10.1145/2556288.2557372
Chong, B., Jayabaskaran, J., Kong, G., Chan, Y. H., Chin, Y. H., Goh, R., Kannan, S., Ng, C. H., Loong, S., Kueh, M. T. W., Lin, C., Anand, V. V., Lee, E. C. Z., Chew, H. S. J., Tan, D. J. H., Chan, K. E., Wang, J. W., Muthiah, M., Dimitriadis, G. K., . . Chew, N. W. S. (2023). Trends and predictions of malnutrition and obesity in 204 countries and territories: An analysis of the Global Burden of Disease Study 2019. *EClinicalMedicine, 57*, 101850. https://doi.org/10.1016/j.eclinm.2023.101850
Chopra, M., & Dasgupta, J. (2021). Concerns of older adults during second COVID wave in India. *Public Health, 17*(10), e057871. https://doi.org/10.1002/alz.057871
Chowdhury, N., Rabel, E. J., Ferraz, D., & del Rio Carral, M. (2025). Between being affected and being an active emotion 'manager': Young women's accounts of social media use and wellbeing. *Psychology & Health*, 1–21. https://doi.org/10.1080/08870446.2025.2474011

Christodoulou, E., Markopoulou, V., & Koutelidakis, A. E. (2024a). Exploring the link between mindful eating, Instagram engagement, and eating disorders: A focus on orthorexia nervosa. *Psychiatry International*, *5*, 27–38. https://doi.org/10.3390/psychiatryint5010003

Christodoulou, N., Laaidi, K., & Geoffroy, P. A. (2024b). Eco-anxiety: Towards a medical model and the new framework of ecolalgia. *Bipolar Disorders*, *26*(6), 532–547. https://doi.org/10.1111/bdi.13446

Chrzan, J., & Cargill, K. (2022). *Anxious eaters: Why we fall for fad diets*. Columbia University Press.

Cianconi, P., Hanife, B., Grillo, F., Betrò, S., Lesmana, C. B. J., & Janiri, L. (2023). Eco-emotions and psychoterratic syndromes: Reshaping mental health assessment under climate change. *Yale Journal of Biology and Medicine*, *96*(2), 211–226. https://doi.org/10.59249/EARX2427

Clark, E. (2022). *Body neutrality: Finding acceptance and liberation in a body-focused culture*. Routledge.

Clayton, S., & Karazsia, B. T. (2020). Development and validation of a measure of climate change anxiety. *Journal of Environmental Psychology*, *69*, 101434. https://doi.org/10.1016/j.jenvp.2020.101434

Cleghorn, E. (2021). *Unwell women: Misdiagnosis and myth in a man-made world*. Dutton.

Cohen, R., Newton-John, T., & Slater, A. (2019). The case for body positivity on social media: Perspectives on current advances and future directions. *Journal of Health Psychology*, *24*(12), 1589–1603. https://doi.org/10.1177/1359105320912450

Coiera, E. (1998). Information epidemics, economics, and immunity on the internet. We still know so little about the effect of information on public health. *British Medical Journal*, *317*(7171), 1469–1470. https://doi.org/10.1136/bmj.317.7171.1469

Collins, J. (2022). Interest in gluten-free foods is hot among Gen Z consumers and QSR diners. *Civic Science*. https://civicscience.com/interest-in-gluten-free-foods-is-hot-among-gen-z-consumers-and-qsr-diners/

Congleton, C., Hölzel, R. K., & Lazar, S. W. (2015). Mindfulness can literally change your brain. *Harvard Business Review*. https://hbr.org/2015/01/mindfulness-can-literally-change-your-brain

Contessa, G. (2023). It takes a village to trust science: Towards a (thoroughly) social approach to public trust in science. *Erkenntnis*, *88*, 2941–2966. https://doi.org/10.1007/s10670-021-00485-8

Cooper, K. (2014). *Obesity: Perception and policy. Multi-country review and survey of policymakers*. European Association for the Study of Obesity.

Costello, A., Abbas, M., Allen, A., Ball, S., Bellamy, R., Friel, S., Groce, N., Johnson, A., Kett, M., Lee, M., Levy, C., Maslin, M., McCoy, D., McGuire, B., Montgomery, H., Napier, D., Pagel, C., Patel, J., de Oliveira, J. A. P., & Redclift, N. (2009). Managing the health effects of climate change. *The Lancet*, *373*(9676), 1693–1733. https://doi.org/10.1016/S0140-6736(09)60935–1

Covino, J. M., Stern, T. W., & Stern, T. A. (2011). Denial of cardiac illness: Consequences and management. *Primary Care Companion for CNS Disorders*, *13*(5), PCC.11f01166. https://doi.org/10.4088/PCC.11f01166

Cox, C., & Fritz, Z. (2022). Presenting complaint: Use of language that disempowers patients. *British Medical Journal*, *377*, e066720. https://doi.org/10.1136/bmj-2021-066720

Cramblitt, B., & Pritchard, M. (2013). Media's influence on the drive for muscularity in undergraduates. *Eating Behaviors*, *14*(4), 441–446. https://doi.org/10.1016/j.eatbeh.2013.08.003

Crampton, C. (2024). *A body made of glass: A cultural history of hypochondria*. Ecco.

Crandall, C. S., & Moriarty, D. (1995). Physical illness stigma and social rejection. *British Journal of Social Psychology*, *34*(Pt 1), 67–83. https://doi.org/10.1111/j.2044-8309.1995.tb01049.x

Crawford, R. (1977). You are dangerous to your health: The ideology and politics of victim blaming. *International Journal of Health Services*, *7*(4), 663–680. https://doi.org/10.2190/YU77-T7B1-EN9X-G0PN

Crawford, R. (1980). Healthism and the medicalization of everyday life. *International Journal of Health Services*, *10*(3), 365–388. https://doi.org/10.2190/3H2H-3XJN-3KAY-G9NY

Crawley, M. (2022). Laboring bodies and the quantified self. *New Genetics and Society*, *41*(1), 66–68. https://doi.org/10.1080/14636778.2022.2029694

Crego, A., Yela, J. R., Gómez-Martínez, M. Á., Riesco-Matías, P., & Petisco-Rodríguez, C. (2021). Relationships between mindfulness, purpose in life, happiness, anxiety, and depression: Testing a mediation model in a sample of women. *International Journal of Environmental Research and Public Health*, *18*(3), 925. https://doi.org/10.3390/ijerph18030925

Creswell, J. D., Welch, W. T., Taylor, S. E., Sherman, D. K., Gruenewald, T. L., & Mann, T. (2005). Affirmation of personal values buffers neuroendocrine and psychological stress responses. *Psychological Science*, *16*(11), 846–851. https://doi.org/10.1111/j.1467-9280.2005.01624.x

Creutzfeldt, C. J., & Holloway, R. G. (2020). Treatment decisions for a future self: Ethical obligations to guide truly informed choices. *JAMA*, *323*(2), 115–116. https://doi.org/10.1001/jama.2019.19652

Cushman, P. (1990). Why the self is empty. Toward a historically situated psychology. *American Psychologist*, *45*(5), 599–611. https://doi.org/10.1037//0003-066x.45.5.599. PMID: 2190505.

Cwynar-Horta, J. (2016). The commodification of the body positive movement on Instagram. *Stream: Interdisciplinary Journal of Communication*, *8*(2), 36–56. https://doi.org/10.21810/strm.v8i2.203

Dane, A., & Bhatia, K. (2023). The social media diet: A scoping review to investigate the association between social media, body image, and eating disorders amongst young people. *PLOS Global Public Health*, *3*(3), e0001091. https://doi.org/10.1371/journal.pgph.0001091

Daniels, K., Fida, R., Stepanek, M., & Gendronneau, C. (2021). Do multicomponent workplace health and wellbeing programs predict changes in health and wellbeing? *International Journal of Environmental Research and Public Health*, *18*(17), 8964. https://doi.org/10.3390/ijerph18178964

Darwin, C. (1998). *The expression of the emotions in man and animals* (P. Ekman, Ed., 3rd ed.). Oxford University Press. (Original work published 1872)

Das, K. P., & Gavade, P. (2024). A review on the efficacy of artificial intelligence for managing anxiety disorders. *Frontiers in Artificial Intelligence*, *7*, 1435895. https://doi.org/10.3389/frai.2024.1435895

Davidson, J. P. (2023). The politics of eco-anxiety: Anthropocene dread from depoliticisation to repoliticisation. *The Anthropocene Review*. https://doi.org/10.1177/20530196231211854

Davison, T. E., McCabe, M. P., Knight, T., & Mellor, D. (2012). Biopsychosocial factors related to depression in aged care residents. *Journal of Affective Disorders*, *142*(1–3), 290–296. https://doi.org/10.1016/j.jad.2012.05.019

De Giglio, O. (2015). Mineral water or tap water? An endless debate. *Annali di Igiene: Medicina Preventiva e di Comunità*, *27*(1), 58–65. https://doi.org/10.7416/ai.2015.2023.

De Lange, C. (2023, September 19). Why being more open about mental health could be making us feel worse. *New Scientist*. https://www.newscientist.com/article/mg25934573–900-why-being-more-open-about-mental-health-could-be-making-us-feel-worse/

De Lemos, S. M. (2016, December). How to overcome your fears. *Oriflame Sweden*. https://hu.oriflame.com/beautyedit/health-beauty/how-to-overcome-your-fears

De Moura Brito Júnior, V., De Magalhães, H. F., & Albuquerque, U. P. (2023). Perception of health risks in contexts of extreme climate change in semiarid northeastern Brazil: An analysis of the role of socioeconomic variables. *Journal of Ethnobiology and Ethnomedicine, 19*, 24. https://doi.org/10.1186/s13002-023-00597-1

de Wit, A., Qu, H., & Bekkers, R. (2022). The health advantage of volunteering is larger for older and less healthy volunteers in Europe: A mega-analysis. *European Journal of Ageing, 19*, 1189–1200. https://doi.org/10.1007/s10433-022-00691-5

Delpino, F. M., da Silva, C. N., Jerônimo, J. S., Mulling, E. S., da Cunha, L. L., Weymar, M. K., Alt, R., Caputo, E. L., & Feter, N. (2022). Prevalence of anxiety during the COVID-19 pandemic: A systematic review and meta-analysis of over 2 million people. *Journal of Affective Disorders, 318*, 272–282. https://doi.org/10.1016/j.jad.2022.09.003

Dennison, L., Morrison, L., Conway, G., & Yardley, L. (2013). Opportunities and challenges for smartphone applications in supporting health behavior change: Qualitative study. *Journal of Medical Internet Research, 15*(4), e86. https://doi.org/10.2196/jmir.2583

Desai, S., & Jena, A. B. (2016). Do celebrity endorsements matter? Observational study of BRCA gene testing and mastectomy rates after Angelina Jolie's New York Times editorial. *British Medical Journal, 355*, i6357. https://doi.org/10.1136/bmj.i6357

DeSteno, D., Petty, R. E., Wegener, D. T., & Rucker, D. D. (2000). Beyond valence in the perception of likelihood: The role of emotion specificity. *Journal of Personality and Social Psychology, 78*(3), 397–416. https://doi.org/10.1037//0022-3514.78.3.397

Díaz Andrade, A., Techatassanasoontorn, A. A., & Singh, H. (2023). Understanding the digital experience: Phenomenological IS research. In R. M. Davison (Ed.), *Handbook of qualitative research methods for information systems* (Chapter 6, pp. 88–103). Edward Elgar Publishing.

Dirksen, S. R. (1995). Search for meaning in long-term cancer survivors. *Journal of Advanced Nursing, 21*(4), 628–633. https://doi.org/10.1046/j.1365-2648.1995.21040628.x

Dobbins, C., & Fairclough, S. (2016). Lifelogging technologies to detect negative emotions associated with cardiovascular disease. In *Applied computing in medicine and health: Emerging topics in computer science and applied computing* (pp. 27–44). https://doi.org/10.1016/B978-0-12-803468-2.00002-3

Dohle, S., Wingen, T., & Baumann, M. (2022). Blaming others for their illness: The influence of health-related implicit theories on blame and social support. *Journal of Applied Social Psychology, 52*(4), 210–219. https://doi.org/10.1111/jasp.12844

Dömötör, Z., Nordin, S., Witthöft, M., & Köteles, F. (2019). Modern health worries: A systematic review. *Journal of Psychosomatic Research, 124*, 109781. https://doi.org/10.1016/j.jpsychores.2019.109781

Dorfmann, M., Menéndez-Blanco, M., & De Angeli, A. (2023). "There is a better you in you": Promises and ideologies of self-tracking technologies. *tripleC: Communication, Capitalism & Critique, 21*(2), 74–91. https://doi.org/10.31269/triplec.v21i2.1411

Doria, M. D. (2006). Bottled water versus tap water: Understanding consumers' preferences. *Journal of Water and Health, 4*(2), 271–276. https://doi.org/10.2166/wh.2006.008

Douglas, M. (1966). *Purity and danger: An analysis of concepts of pollution and taboo*. Routledge & Kegan Paul.

Douglas, M. (1982). *Essays in the sociology of perception*. Routledge & Keagan Paul.

Douglas, M. (1992). *Risk and blame: Essays in cultural theory*. Routledge.

Douglas, M., & Wildavsky, A. (1982). *Risk and culture: An essay on the selection of technological and environmental dangers*. University of California Press.

Drotner, K. (1999). Dangerous media? Panic discourses and dilemmas of modernity. *Paedagogica Historica, 35*(3), 593–619. https://doi.org/10.1080/0030923990350303

Druss, B. G., & Marcus, S. C. (2004). Use of psychotropic medications before and after Sept. 11, 2001. *American Journal of Psychiatry, 161*(8), 1377–1387. https://doi.org/10.1176/appi.ajp.161.8.1377

Dumitrescu, A., Dogaru, C. B., Duta, C., Zetu, L., & Zetu, I. (2014). The inter-relationships between body dissatisfaction, body image disturbance, and oral health. *Procedia – Social and Behavioral Sciences, 127*, 368–372. https://doi.org/10.1016/j.sbspro.2014.03.273

Dunbar, R. I. M. (2017). Breaking bread: The functions of social eating. *Adaptive Human Behavior and Physiology, 3,* 198–211. https://doi.org/10.1007/s40750-017-0061-4
Duncan, C., & Cacciatore, J. (2015). A systematic review of the peer-reviewed literature on self-blame, guilt, and shame. *Omega (Westport), 71*(4), 312–342. https://doi.org/10.1177/0030222815572604
Durbhakula, S., & Fortin, A. H. (2023). Turning down the flame on medical gaslighting. *Journal of General Internal Medicine, 38*(12), 3426–3427. https://doi.org/10.1007/s11606-023-08302-4
Durkheim, É. (1982). *The rules of sociological method.* Simon and Schuster. (Original work published 1895)
Dweck, C. S. (2000). *Self-theories: Their role in motivation, personality, and development.* Psychology Press.
Editorial. (2024, April 10). What happens when climate change and the mental-health crisis collide? *Nature, 628,* 235. https://doi.org/10.1038/d41586-024-00993-x
Elhai, J. D., McKay, D., Yang, H., Minaya, C., Montag, C., & Asmundson, G. J. G. (2021). Health anxiety related to problematic smartphone use and gaming disorder severity during COVID-19: Fear of missing out as a mediator. *Human Behavior & Emerging Technologies, 3,* 137–146. https://doi.org/10.1002/hbe2.227
Elias, N. (2000). *The civilizing process: Sociogenetic and psychogenetic investigations* (Rev. ed.). Blackwell.
Elliott, A. (2024). *Algorithms of anxiety: Fear in the digital age.* Polity.
Erikson, E. H. (1956). The problem of ego identity. *Journal of the American Psychoanalytic Association, 4*(1), 56–121. https://doi.org/10.1177/000306515600400104
Eriksson, M., Ekström-Bergström, A., Arvidsson, S., Jormfeldt, H., Thorstensson, S., Åström, U., Lundgren, I., & Roxberg, Å. (2024). Meaning of wellness in caring science based on Rodgers's evolutionary concept analysis. *Scandinavian Journal of the Caring Sciences, 38*(1), 185–199. https://doi.org/10.1111/scs.13196
Eunsoo, C., Chentsova-Dutton, Y., & Parrott, G. W. (2016). The effectiveness of somatization in communicating distress in Korean and American cultural contexts. *Frontiers in Psychology, 7,* 383. https://doi.org/10.3389/fpsyg.2016.00383
Eurostat. (2022, December 15). What did we use the internet for in 2022? *Eurostat News.* https://ec.europa.eu/eurostat/web/main/news/articles
Ezeudoka, B. C., & Fan, M. (2024). Exploring the impact of digital distrust on user resistance to e-health services among older adults: The moderating effect of anticipated regret. *Humanities and Social Sciences Communications, 11,* 1190. https://doi.org/10.1057/s41599-024-02793-x
Falk, P. (1994). *The consuming body.* Sage Publications.
Fang, S., & Mushtaque, I. (2024). The moderating role of health literacy and health-promoting behavior in the relationship among health anxiety, emotional regulation, and cyberchondria. *Psychology Research and Behavior Management, 17,* 51–62. https://doi.org/10.2147/PRBM.S446448
Fawcett, B., Weber, Z., & Bannister, H. (2020). *The medicalisation of everyday life: A critical perspective.* Bloomsbury Publishing.
Featherstone, M., Hepworth, M., & Turner, B. S. (1991). *The body: Social process and cultural theory.* Sage.
Feng, S., Mäntymäki, M., Dhir, A., & Salmela, H. (2021). How self-tracking and the quantified self promote health and well-being: Systematic review. *Journal of Medical Internet Research, 23*(9), e25171. https://doi.org/10.2196/25171
Ferreira, K. B., & Webber, K. T. (2023). The politics of 'obesity': Medicalization, stigmatization and liberation of fat bodies. In M. Halliwell & S. A. Jones (Eds.), *The Edinburgh companion to the politics of American health* (pp. 149–166). Cambridge University Press. https://doi.org/10.1017/9781009387673.009
Fielding, S. (2022, October 12). A critical look at self-care culture and the importance of knowing its limits. *VeryWellMind.* https://www.verywellmind.com/a-critical-look-at-self-care-culture-6743663

Finucane, M. L. (2000). The affect heuristic in judgement of risks and benefits. *Journal of Behavioral Decision Making, 13*(1), 1–17. https://doi.org/10.1002/(SICI)1099-0771(200001/03)13:1<1::AID-BDM333>3.0.CO;2-S

Fischer, L. B. (Ed.). (2024). *Routledge handbook of risk, crisis, and disaster communication*. Routledge.

Fiske, A., Buyx, A., & Prainsack, B. (2019). Health information counselors: A new profession for the age of big data. *Academic Medicine, 94*(1), 37–41. https://doi.org/10.1097/ACM.0000000000002395

Fitzgerald, H. E., Lubin, R. E., Duncan, T., Hiserodt, M., & Otto, M. W. (2022). Underscoring the F in FoMO: How does anxiety sensitivity contribute to fear of missing out? *Cognitive Behaviour Therapy, 52*(1), 38–46. https://doi.org/10.1080/16506073.2022.2131619

Fitzpatrick, P. J. (2023). Improving health literacy using the power of digital communications to achieve better health outcomes for patients and practitioners. *Frontiers in Digital Health, 5*, 1264780. https://doi.org/10.3389/fdgth.2023.1264780

Fleary, S. A., Joseph, P. L., Gonçalves, C., Somogie, J., & Angeles, J. (2022). The relationship between health literacy and mental health attitudes and beliefs. *HLRP: Health Literacy Research and Practice, 6*(4), e270–e279. https://doi.org/10.3928/24748307-20221018-01

Fortune Business Insights. (2022). *The global gluten-free food market is projected to grow from $5.72 billion in 2021 to $9.99 billion in 2028 at a CAGR of 8.29% in forecast period, 2021–2028. Market research report*. https://fortunebusinessinsights.com

Foucault, M. (1988). Technologies of the self. In L. H. Martin, H. Gutman, & P. H. Hutton (Eds.), *Technologies of the self: A seminar with Michel Foucault* (pp. 16–30). Tavistock Publications.

Foucault, M. (2008). *The birth of biopolitics: Lectures at the Collège de France 1978–1979* (G. Bucknell, Trans.). Palgrave Macmillan.

Foulkes, L., & Andrews, J. L. (2023). Are mental health awareness efforts contributing to the rise in reported mental health problems? A call to test the prevalence inflation hypothesis. *New Ideas in Psychology, 69*, 1–6. https://doi.org/10.1016/j.newideapsych.2023.101010

Fox, N., & Ward, K. J. (2008). You are what you eat? Vegetarianism, health, and identity. *Social Science & Medicine, 66*(12), 2585–2595. https://doi.org/10.1016/j.socscimed.2008.02.011

Frances, A. (2013). *Saving normal: An insider's revolt against out-of-control psychiatric diagnosis, DSM-5, Big Pharma, and the medicalization of ordinary life*. William Morrow & Co.

Frankl, V. (1988). *The will to meaning: Foundations and applications of logotherapy*. New American Library.

Frankl, V. E. (2021). *Man's search for meaning: An introduction to logotherapy* (6th ed.). Rider. (Original work published 1946)

Freeman, H. J. (2015). Celiac disease: A disorder emerging from antiquity, its evolving classification and risk, and potential new treatment paradigms. *Gut Liver, 9*(1), 28–37. https://doi.org/10.5009/gnl14288.

Freud, S. (1989). *Totem and taboo*. W. W. Norton. (Original work published 1913)

Freud, S. (1990). *Five lectures on psycho-analysis* (Standard ed.). W. W. Norton & Company. (Original work published 1909)

Freud, S. (2002). *Civilization and its discontents*. Penguin. (Original work published 1930)

Freud, S., & Breuer, J. (2004). *Studies in hysteria* (N. Luckhurst, Trans.). Penguin Books. (Original work published 1895)

The Frisky. (2010, March 2). Feasting on nothing: French women go crazy for the 'Air Diet'. *Yahoo! Life*. https://www.yahoo.com/lifestyle/tagged/health/healthy-living/feasting-on-nothing-french-women-go-crazy-for-the-quot-air-diet-quot–982317.html

Fuławka, K., Hertwig, R., & Pachur, T. (2024). COVID-19 vaccine refusal is driven by deliberate ignorance and cognitive distortions. *npj Vaccines, 9*, 167. https://doi.org/10.1038/s41541-024-00951-8

Furedi, F. (2007). *Culture of fear revisited: Risk-taking and the morality of low expectation*. Continuum.

Gale, J. (2021). Secular mindfulness and its relationship to mental health: Benefits, McMindfulness and other critiques, and mindfulness revisited. In J. N. Lester & M. O'Reilly (Eds.), *The Palgrave Encyclopedia of Critical Perspectives on Mental Health*. Palgrave Macmillan. https://doi.org/10.1007/978-3-030-12852-4_47-1

Gardiner, G., Lee, D., Baranski, E., & Funder, D. (2020). Members of the international situations project. Happiness around the world: A combined etic-emic approach across 63 countries. *PLoS ONE, 15*(12), e0242718. https://doi.org/10.1371/journal.pone.0242718

Gefen, D. (2017). *The self-help addict: Turn an overdose of information into a life of transformation*. CreateSpace Independent Publishing Platform.

George, J. F. (2024). Discovering why people believe disinformation about healthcare. *PLoS ONE, 19*(3), e0300497. https://doi.org/10.1371/journal.pone.0300497

Gianfredi, V., Mazziotta, F., Clerici, G., Astorri, E., Oliani, F., Cappellina, M., Catalini, A., Dell'Osso, B. M., Pregliasco, F. E., Castaldi, S., & Benatti, B. (2024). Climate change perception and mental health: Results from a systematic review of the literature. *European Journal of Investigation in Health, Psychology and Education, 14*(1), 215–229. https://doi.org/10.3390/ejihpe14010014

Gibson, P. R., Skodje, G. I., & Lundin, K. E. (2017). Non-coeliac gluten sensitivity. *Journal of Gastroenterology and Hepatology, 32*(Suppl 1), 86–89. https://doi.org/10.1111/jgh.13705

Gigerenzer, G. (2014). *Risk savvy: How to make good decisions*. Viking Penguin.

Gillen, M. M. (2015). Associations between positive body image and indicators of men's and women's mental and physical health. *Body Image, 13*, 67–74. https://doi.org/10.1016/j.bodyim.2015.01.002

Gilman, S., King, H., Porter, R., Rousseau, R. S., & Showalter, E. (1993). *Hysteria beyond Freud*. University of California Press.

Giritli-Nygren, K., & Olofsson, A. (2014). Intersectional approaches in health risk research: A critical review. *Sociology Compass, 8*(9), 1112–1126. https://doi.org/10.1111/soc4.12176

Goddard, E. (2024, July 1). Self-help was meant to make me feel better. Instead, it turned toxic – and borderline dangerous. *The Guardian*. https://www.theguardian.com/commentisfree/article/2024/jul/01/self-help-toxic-books-courses-apps

Goh, P. H., Loh, H. Y., Chung, K. R., & Ramadas, A. (2024). Body (dis)satisfaction and health screening behaviors: A systematic review of observational studies. *Journal of Health Psychology, 29*(2), 137–155. https://doi.org/10.1177/13591053231189413

Golden, B. (2024, June 2). Self-compassion reduces stigma in chronic physical illness. *Psychology Today*. https://www.psychologytoday.com/intl/blog/overcoming-destructive-anger/202406/self-compassion-reduces-stigma-in-chronic-physical-illness

Goldware, K. (2022, April 8). #DiagnosisFat: When doctors ignore real problems. *The College Voice*. https://www.mcccvoice.org/diagnosisfat/

Gonzalez, B. D., Jim, H. S., Cessna, J. M., Small, B. J., Sutton, S. K., & Jacobsen, P. B. (2015). Concealment of lung cancer diagnosis: Prevalence and correlates. *Psycho-Oncology, 24*(12), 1774–1783. https://doi.org/10.1002/pon.3793

González Ramírez, M. L., García Vázquez, J. P., Rodríguez, M. D., Padilla-López, L. A., Galindo-Aldana, G. M., & Cuevas-González, D. (2023). Wearables for stress management: A scoping review. *Healthcare, 11*(17), 2369. https://doi.org/10.3390/healthcare11172369

Goonesekera, Y., & Donkin, L. (2022). A cognitive behavioral therapy chatbot (Otis) for health anxiety management: Mixed methods pilot study. *JMIR Formative Research, 6*(10), e37877. https://doi.org/10.2196/37877

Grassi, L., Caruso, R., Sabato, S., Massarenti, S., Nanni, M. G., & The UniFe Psychiatry Working Group Coauthors. (2015). Psychosocial screening and assessment in oncology and palliative care settings. *Frontiers in Psychology, 5*, 1485. https://doi.org/10.3389/fpsyg.2014.01485

Greco, M. (1993). Psychosomatic subjects and the 'duty to be well': Personal agency within medical rationality. *Economy and Society*, *22*(3), 357–372. https://doi.org/10.1080/03085149300000024

Greco, M. (1998). *Illness as a work of thought: A Foucauldian perspective on psychosomatics*. Routledge.

Greville-Harris, M., Talbot, C. V., Moseley, R. L., & Vuillier, L. (2022). Conceptualisations of health in orthorexia nervosa: A mixed-methods study. *Eating and Weight Disorders*, *27*, 3135–3143. https://doi.org/10.1007/s40519-022-01443-1

Groopman, J. (2003, August 11). Sick with worry: Can hypochondria be cured? *The New Yorker*, 28–34. https://www.newyorker.com/magazine/2003/08/11/treating-hypochondria

Grosso, F., Barbiani, D., Cavalera, C., Volpato, E., & Pagnini, F. (2024). Risk factors associated with nocebo effects: A review of reviews. *Brain, Behavior & Immunity – Health*, *38*, 100800. https://doi.org/10.1016/j.bbih.2024.100800

Guillaud, A., Allenet, B., & Pinsault, N. (2020). Does dissatisfaction with physicians lead patients to alternative practitioners? *Complementary Therapies in Clinical Practice*, *39*, 101109. https://doi.org/10.1016/j.ctcp.2020.101109

Gulseven, O., & Wohlgenant, M. (2017). What are the factors affecting the consumers' milk choices? *Agricultural Economics*, *63*, 271–282. https://doi.org/10.17221/335/2015-AGRICECON

Gunderman, R. (2000). Illness as failure: Blaming patients. *The Hastings Center Report*, *30*(4), 7–11. https://doi.org/10.2307/3527639

Gwynne, A. E. (2024). 'Up to you': Self-help books, depression, and the reconstruction of reading. *Media, Culture & Society*, *46*(2), 324–342. https://doi.org/10.1177/01634437231198431

Hacker, K. (2024). The burden of chronic disease. *Mayo Clinic Proceedings: Innovations, Quality & Outcomes*, *8*(1), 112–119. https://doi.org/10.1016/j.mayocpiqo.2023.08.005

Halding, A. G., Heggdal, K., & Wahl, A. (2011). Experiences of self-blame and stigmatisation for self-infliction among individuals living with COPD. *Scandinavian Journal of Caring Sciences*, *25*(1), 100–107. https://doi.org/10.1111/j.1471-6712.2010.00796.x

Halliwell, E., Jarman, H., Tylka, T., & Slater, A. (2017). Adapting the Body Appreciation Scale-2 for children: A psychometric analysis of the BAS-2C. *Body Image*, *21*, 97–102. https://doi.org/10.1016/j.bodyim.2017.03.005

Hampel, J. (2006). Different concepts of risk: A challenge for risk communication. *International Journal of Medical Microbiology*, *296*(Suppl. 40), 5–10. https://doi.org/10.1016/j.ijmm.2005.12.002

Hamrick, L. (2023). Artificial intimacy: Virtual friends, digital lovers, algorithmic matchmakers. *AI & Society*. Advance online publication. https://doi.org/10.1007/s00146-022-01624-7

Han, B.-C. (2021). *The palliative society: Pain today*. Polity Press.

Hancı, E., Ruijten, P. A. M., Lacroix, J., & IJsselsteijn, W. A. (2021). The impact of mindset on self-tracking experience. *Frontiers in Digital Health*, *3*, 676742. https://doi.org/10.3389/fdgth.2021.676742

Hanganu-Bresch, C. (2020). Orthorexia: Eating right in the context of healthism. *Medical Humanities*, *46*(3), 311–322. https://doi.org/10.1136/medhum-2019-011681

Hannah, K., Marie, K., Olaf, H., Stephan, B., Andreas, D., Wilson Michael, L., Till, B., & Peter, D. (2023). The global economic burden of health anxiety/hypochondriasis: A systematic review. *BMC Public Health*, *23*, 2237. https://doi.org/10.1186/s12889-023-17159-5

Hansson, K. (2020). Critical places and emerging health matters: Body, risk, and spatial obstacles. In S. Atkinson & R. Hunt (Eds.), *GeoHumanities and Health* (pp. 71–83). Springer. https://doi.org/10.1007/978-3-030-21406-7_5

Haque, M. D. R., & Rubya, S. (2023). An overview of chatbot-based mobile mental health apps: Insights from app description and user reviews. *JMIR mHealth and uHealth*, *11*, e44838. https://doi.org/10.2196/44838

Hardey, M. M. (2022). Tracking the trackers: Self-tracking in households as social practice. *Digital Health, 8*, 20552076221093131. https://doi.org/10.1177/20552076221093131

Harry, K. M., Bennett, K. K., Clark, J. M., Howarter, A. D., & Eways, K. R. (2015). Self-blame attributions and cardiac symptom experiences in cardiac rehabilitation patients: A preliminary study. *North American Journal of Psychology, 17*(3), 541.

Hart, T., Hanks, R., Bogner, J. A., Millis, S., & Esselman, P. (2007). Blame attribution in intentional and unintentional traumatic brain injury: Longitudinal changes and impact on subjective well-being. *Rehabilitation Psychology, 52*(2), 152–161. https://doi.org/10.1037/0090-5550.52.2.152

Harwood, T. M., & L'Abate, L. (2010). *Self-help in mental health: A critical review*. Springer.

Haslam, N., & Tse, J. S. (2024). Public awareness of mental illness: Mental health literacy or concept creep? *Australasian Psychiatry*. https://doi.org/10.1177/10398562241292202

Hassan, H. F., Mourad, L., Khatib, N., Assi, R., Akil, S., El Khatib, S., & Hteit, R. (2024). Perceptions towards gluten-free products among consumers: A narrative review. *Applied Food Research, 2*, 100441. https://doi.org/10.1016/j.afres.2024.100441

Hathaway, J., & Maibach, E. W. (2018). Health implications of climate change: A review of the literature about the perception of the public and health professionals. *Current Environmental Health Reports, 5*(3), 197–204. https://doi.org/10.1007/s40572-018-0190-3

Hazzard, V. M., Telke, S. E., Simone, M., Anderson, L. M., Larson, N. I., & Neumark-Sztainer, D. (2021). Intuitive eating longitudinally predicts better psychological health and lower use of disordered eating behaviors: Findings from EAT 2010–2018. *Eating and Weight Disorders, 26*(1), 287–294. https://doi.org/10.1007/s40519-020-00852-4

Heath, S. (2011). Hypochondria: Medical condition, creative malady. *Brain, 134*(4), 1244–1249. https://doi.org/10.1093/brain/awr006

Heelas, P. (1998). Emotion talk across cultures. In R. Harré (Ed.), *The social construction of emotion* (pp. 234–266). Blackwell.

Hefferon, K. (2015). The role of embodiment in optimal functioning. In S. Joseph (Ed.), *Positive psychology in practice: Promoting human flourishing in work, health, education, and everyday life* (pp. 791–805). John Wiley & Sons Inc.

Hefferon, K., Grealy, M., & Mutrie, N. (2009). Post-traumatic growth and life-threatening physical illness: A systematic review of the qualitative literature. *British Journal of Health Psychology, 14*(2), 343–378. https://doi.org/10.1348/135910708X332936

Helm, P. J., Jimenez, T., Galgali, M. S., Edwards, M. E., Vail, K. E., III, & Arndt, J. (2022). Divergent effects of social media use on meaning in life via loneliness and existential isolation during the coronavirus pandemic. *Journal of Social and Personal Relationships, 39*(6), 1768–1793. https://doi.org/10.1177/02654075211066922

Hendl, T., & Shukla, A. (2024). Can digital health democratize health care? *Bioethics, 38*(6), 491–502. https://doi.org/10.1111/bioe.13266

Herbener, A. B., & Damholdt, M. F. (2025). Are lonely youngsters turning to chatbots for companionship? The relationship between chatbot usage and social connectedness in Danish high-school students. *International Journal of Human-Computer Studies, 196*, 103409. https://doi.org/10.1016/j.ijhcs.2024.103409

Hickman, C., Marks, E., Pihkala, P., Clayton, S., Lewandowski, R. E., Mayall, E. E., Wray, B., Mellor, C., & van Susteren, L. (2021). Climate anxiety in children and young people and their beliefs about government responses to climate change: A global survey. *The Lancet Planetary Health, 5*(12), e863–e873. https://doi.org/10.1016/S2542-5196(21)00278-3

Hirschlag, A. (2020, August 10). COVID-19 is making everybody's cyberchondria worse. *ELLE*. https://www.elle.com/life-love/a33482294/covid-19-cyberchondria-webmd/

Hjorth, L., Ohashi, K., Sinanan, J., Horst, H., Pink, S., Kato, F., & Zhou, B. (2020). *Digital media practices in households: Kinship through data*. Amsterdam University Press.

Ho, S. M. Y., & Cheng, C. T. (2023). Illusory versus constructive posttraumatic growth in cancer. In R. Berger (Ed.), *The Routledge international handbook of posttraumatic growth* (pp. xx–xx). Routledge. https://doi.org/10.4324/9781032208688-4

Höffken, O. (2024). Critical theory and human nature: Hartmut Rosa's resonance theory from an evolutionary-anthropological perspective. *Acta Academica*, *56*(2), 116–137. https://doi.org/10.38140/aa.v56i2.8975

Hogg, T. L., Stanley, S. K., O'Brien, L. V., Wilson, M. S., & Watsford, C. R. (2021). The Hogg eco-anxiety scale: Development and validation of a multidimensional scale. *Global Environmental Change, 71,* 102391. https://doi.org/10.1016/j.gloenvcha.2021.102391

Høgset, K., Olin, M., & Wallin, E. (Directors). (2020). *Self portrait* [Film]. Speranza Film.

Horney, K. (1937). *The neurotic personality of our time*. W. W. Norton & Company.

Hornsey, M. J. (2020). Why facts are not enough: Understanding and managing the motivated rejection of science. *Current Directions in Psychological Science*, *29*(6), 583–591. https://doi.org/10.1177/0963721420969364

Horovitz, O., & Argyrides, M. (2023). Orthorexia and orthorexia nervosa: A comprehensive examination of prevalence, risk factors, diagnosis, and treatment. *Nutrients*, *15*(17), 3851. https://doi.org/10.3390/nu15173851

Hrehorów, E., Salomon, J., Matusiak, L., Reich, A., & Szepietowski, J. C. (2012). Patients with psoriasis feel stigmatized. *Acta Dermatologica Venereologica*, *92*(1), 67–72. https://doi.org/10.2340/00015555-1193

Huang, Y., & Zhao, N. (2021). Mental health burden for the public affected by the COVID-19 outbreak in China: Who will be the high-risk group? *Psychology, Health & Medicine*, *26*(1), 23–34. https://doi.org/10.1080/13548506.2020.1754438

Huang, Z., Yu, T., Wu, S., & Hu, A. (2021). Correlates of stigma for patients with cancer: A systematic review and meta-analysis. *Supportive Care in Cancer, 29,* 1195–1203. https://doi.org/10.1007/s00520-020-05780-8

Huhn, S., Axt, M., Gunga, H. C., Maggioni, M. A., Munga, S., Obor, D., Sié, A., Boudo, V., Bunker, A., Sauerborn, R., Bärnighausen, T., & Barteit, S. (2022). The impact of wearable technologies in health research: Scoping review. *JMIR mHealth and uHealth, 10*(1), e34384. https://doi.org/10.2196/34384

Humphrey, L., Clifford, D., & Neyman Morris, M. (2015). Health at Every Size college course reduces dieting behaviors and improves intuitive eating, body esteem, and anti-fat attitudes. *Journal of Nutrition Education and Behavior*, *47*(4), 354–360.e1. https://doi.org/10.1016/j.jneb.2015.01.008

Humphreys, L. (2018). *The qualified self. Social media and the accounting of everyday life.* The MIT Press.

Hunter, K. M. (1990). An N of 1: Syndrome letters in *The New England Journal of Medicine*. *Perspectives in Biology and Medicine*, *33*(2), 237–251. https://doi.org/10.1353/pbm.1990.0028

Hunter, K. M. (2020). *Doctors' stories: The narrative structure of medical knowledge*. Princeton University Press.

Hyland, T. (2015). McMindfulness in the workplace: Vocational learning and the commodification of the present moment. *Journal of Vocational Education & Training*, *65*(2), 219–234. https://doi.org/10.1080/13636820.2015.1022871

Infurna, F. J., & Jayawickreme, E. (2021). Redesigning research on post-traumatic growth: Current knowledge and new directions. In F. J. Infurna & E. Jayawickreme (Eds.), *Redesigning research on post-traumatic growth: Challenges, pitfalls, and new directions* (pp. 280–296). Oxford University Press.

IPSOS. (2022, November 24). Internet users' trust in the Internet has dropped significantly since 2019. *Technology & Telecom*. https://www.ipsos.com/en/trust-in-the-internet-2022

Jackson, D. (2023, January 13). Kourtney Kardashian, Jessica Alba and more celebrities who are gluten-free. *Us Weekly*. https://www.usmagazine.com/food/pictures/celebrities-who-follow-gluten-free-diets/

Jackson, S. J., Sam, M. P., Dawson, M. C., & Porter, D. (2022). The wellbeing pandemic: Outline of a contested terrain and a proposed research agenda. *Frontiers in Sociology*, *7*, 950557. https://doi.org/10.3389/fsoc.2022.950557

Jacobsen, M. H. (2021). Fear and retrotopia: Critical reflections on the rise of defensive emotions in liquid modernity. *Zoon Politikon, 12*, 94–124. https://doi.org/10.4467/2543408XZOP.21.003.14426
Jadhakhan, F., Romeu, D., Lindner, O., Blakemore, A., & Guthrie, E. (2022). Prevalence of medically unexplained symptoms in adults who are high users of healthcare services and magnitude of associated costs: A systematic review. *BMJ Open, 12*(10), e059971. https://doi.org/10.1136/bmjopen-2021-059971
Jannati, Y., Nia, H. S., Froelicher, E. S., Goudarzian, A. H., & Yaghoobzadeh, A. (2020). Self-blame attributions of patients: A systematic review study. *Central Asian Journal of Global Health, 9*(1), e419. https://doi.org/10.5195/cajgh.2020.419
Janoff-Bulman, R. (1992). *Shattered assumptions: Towards a new psychology of trauma.* The Free Press.
Jarvis, D. S. L. (2007). Risk, globalisation and the state: A critical appraisal of Ulrich Beck and the world risk society thesis. *Global Society, 21*(1), 23–46. https://doi.org/10.1080/13600820601116468
Javaid, S. F., Hashim, I. J., Hashim, M. J., Stip, E., Samad, M. A., & Ahbabi, A. A. (2023). Epidemiology of anxiety disorders: Global burden and sociodemographic associations. *Middle East Current Psychiatry, 30*(44). https://doi.org/10.1186/s43045-023-00315-3
Jay, M., Kalet, A., Ark, T., McMacken, M., Messito, M. J., Richter, R., Schlair, S., Sherman, S., Zabar, S., & Gillespie, C. (2009). Physicians' attitudes about obesity and their associations with competency and specialty: A cross-sectional study. *BMC Health Services Research, 9*, 106. https://doi.org/10.1186/1472-6963-9-106
Jerath, R., Syam, M., & Ahmed, S. (2023). The future of stress management: Integration of smartwatches and HRV technology. *Sensors, 23*(17), 7314. https://doi.org/10.3390/s23177314
Jiao, W., Chang, A., Ho, M., Lu, Q., Liu, M. T., & Schulz, P. J. (2023). Predicting and empowering health for Generation Z by comparing health information seeking and digital health literacy: Cross-sectional questionnaire study. *Journal of Medical Internet Research, 25*, e47595. https://doi.org/10.2196/47595
Jolie, A. (2013, May 13). My medical choice. *The New York Times*. https://www.nytimes.com/2013/05/14/opinion/my-medical-choice.html
Jolie Pitt, A. (2015, March 24). Diary of a surgery. *The New York Times*. https://www.nytimes.com/2015/03/24/opinion/angelina-jolie-pitt-diary-of-a-surgery.html
Jones, A. L. (2017). The gluten-free diet: Fad or necessity? *Diabetes Spectrum, 30*(2), 118–123. https://doi.org/10.2337/ds16-0022
Jones, R. (2020, October 26). Why food allergies are on the rise? *BBC*. https://www.bbc.com/future/article/20201023-food-allergies-why-nut-dairy-and-food-allergy-are-rising
Jordanova, L. (1993). Gender and the historiography of science. *The British Journal for the History of Science, 26*(4), 469–483. http://www.jstor.org/stable/4027467
Joseph, S. (2013). *What doesn't kill us: The new psychology of posttraumatic growth*. Basic Books.
Jungmann, S. M., Gropalis, M., Schenkel, S. K., & Witthöft, M. (2024). Is cyberchondria specific to hypochondriasis? *Journal of Anxiety Disorders, 102*, 102798. https://doi.org/10.1016/j.janxdis.2023.102798
Jungmann, S. M., & Witthöft, M. (2020). Health anxiety, cyberchondria, and coping in the current COVID-19 pandemic: Which factors are related to coronavirus anxiety? *Journal of Anxiety Disorders, 73*, 102239. https://doi.org/10.1016/j.janxdis.2020.102239
Kabat-Zinn, J. (2003). Mindfulness-based interventions in context: Past, present, and future. *Clinical Psychology: Science and Practice, 10*(2), 144–156. https://doi.org/10.1093/clipsy.bpg016
Kahneman, D., & Deaton, A. (2010). High income improves evaluation of life but not emotional well-being. *Proceedings of the National Academy of Sciences, 107*, 16489–16493. https://doi.org/10.1073/pnas.1011492107

Kanazawa, S. (2020). Does global warming contribute to the obesity epidemic? *Environmental Research, 182*, 108962. https://doi.org/10.1016/j.envres.2019.108962

Kapeller, A. (2024). Phenomenology and empowerment in self-testing apps. *Bioethics, 38*(9), 770–777. https://doi.org/10.1111/bioe.13293

Kapeller, A., & Loosman, I. (2023). Empowerment through health self-testing apps? Revisiting empowerment as a process. *Medicine, Health Care and Philosophy, 26*(1), 143–152. https://doi.org/10.1007/s11019-022-10132-w

Kaplan, J. (2019). Self-care as self-blame redux: Stress as personal and political. *Kennedy Institute of Ethics Journal, 29*(2), 97–123. https://doi.org/10.1353/ken.2019.0017

Karayigit, C., Ozier, M., Bloom, A., Weaver, M., & Wiltz, S. (2024). Meaning in life among emerging adults: An examination of gender, relationship status, and social media use. *The Journal of Humanistic Counseling*. https://doi.org/10.1002/johc.12222

Karkosz, S., Szymański, R., Sanna, K., & Michałowski, J. (2024). Effectiveness of a web-based and mobile therapy chatbot on anxiety and depressive symptoms in subclinical young adults: Randomized controlled trial. *JMIR Formative Research, 8*, e47960. https://doi.org/10.2196/47960

Kellner, R. (1987). *Somatization and hypochondriasis*. Praeger.

Kent, R. (2018). Social media and self-tracking: Representing the 'health self'. In B. Ajana (Ed.), *Self-tracking: Empirical and philosophical investigations* (pp. 61–77). Palgrave Macmillan.

Kent, R. (2020). Self-tracking health over time: From the use of Instagram to perform optimal health to the protective shield of the digital detox. *Social Media + Society, 6*(3). https://doi.org/10.1177/2056305120940694

Kenyon, F. E. (1966). Hypochondriasis: A survey of some historical, clinical and social aspects. *International Journal of Psychiatry, 2*(3), 308–334. PMID: 5327325.

Kerr, G. R., Wu-Lee, M., El-Lozy, M., McGandy, R., & Stare, F. J. (1977). Objectivity of food-symptomatology surveys: Questionnaire on the "Chinese Restaurant Syndrome." *Journal of the American Dietetic Association, 71*, 263–268. PMID: 886129.

Kerr, G. R., Wu-Lee, M., El-Lozy, M., McGandy, R., & Stare, F. J. (1979). Food-symptomatology questionnaires: Risks of demand-bias questions and population-biased surveys. In L. J. Filer, S. Garattini, M. R. Kare, W. A. Reynolds, & R. J. Wurtman (Eds.), *Glutamic acid: Advances in biochemistry and physiology* (pp. 375–387). Raven Press.

Khan, S. S., Ning, H., Sinha, A., Wilkins, J., Allen, N. B., Vu, T. H. T., Berry, J. D., Lloyd-Jones, D. M., & Sweis, R. (2021). Cigarette smoking and competing risks for fatal and nonfatal cardiovascular disease subtypes across the life course. *Journal of the American Heart Association, 10*(23), e021751. https://doi.org/10.1161/JAHA.121.021751

Khawaja, Z., & Bélisle-Pipon, J. C. (2023). Your robot therapist is not your therapist: Understanding the role of AI-powered mental health chatbots. *Frontiers in Digital Health, 5*, 1278186. https://doi.org/10.3389/fdgth.2023.1278186

Kholeif, O. (Ed.). (2021). *Art in the age of anxiety*. The MIT Press.

Khosravi, M., Izadi, R., & Azar, G. (2024). Factors influencing the engagement with electronic mental health technologies: A systematic review of reviews. *Administration and Policy in Mental Health and Mental Health Services Research*. https://doi.org/10.1007/s10488-024-01420-z

Khoury, B., Sharma, M., Rush, S. E., & Fournier, C. (2015). Mindfulness-based stress reduction for healthy individuals: A meta-analysis. *Journal of Psychosomatic Research, 78*(6), 519–528. https://doi.org/10.1016/j.jpsychores.2015.03.009

Kierkegaard, S. (1959). *Either/or*. Doubleday. (Original work published 1843)

Kierkegaard, S. (2015). *The concept of anxiety: A simple psychologically oriented deliberation in view of the dogmatic problem of hereditary sin* (A. Hannay, Trans.). Liveright. (Original work published 1844)

Kiknadze, N. C., & Fowers, B. J. (2023). Cultural variation in flourishing. *Journal of Happiness Studies: An Interdisciplinary Forum on Subjective Well-Being, 24*(7), 2223–2244. https://doi.org/10.1007/s10902-023-00677-9

Kim, E. S., Chen, Y., Nakamura, J. S., Ryff, C. D., & VanderWeele, T. J. (2022). Sense of purpose in life and subsequent physical, behavioral, and psychosocial health: An outcome-wide approach. *American Journal of Health Promotion*, *36*(1), 137–147. https://doi.org/10.1177/08901171211038545

Kim, E. S., Shiba, K., Boehm, J. K., & Kubzansky, L. D. (2020). Sense of purpose in life and five health behaviors in older adults. *Preventive Medicine*, *139*, 106172. https://doi.org/10.1016/j.ypmed.2020.106172

Kington, R. S., Arnesen, S., Chou, W. S., Curry, S. J., Lazer, D., & Villarruel, A. M. (2021). Identifying credible sources of health information in social media: Principles and attributes. *NAM Perspectives*. https://doi.org/10.31478/202107a

Király, O., Potenza, M. N., Stein, D. J., King, D. L., Hodgins, D. C., Saunders, J. B., Griffiths, M. D., Gjoneska, B., Billieux, J., Brand, M., Abbott, M. W., Chamberlain, S. R., Corazza, O., Burkauskas, J., Sales, C. M. D., Montag, C., Lochner, C., Grünblatt, E., Wegmann, E., Martinotti, G., . . . Lee, H. K. (2020). Preventing problematic internet use during the COVID-19 pandemic: Consensus guidance. *Comprehensive Psychiatry*, *100*, 152180. https://doi.org/10.1016/j.comppsych.2020.152180

Kirmayer, L. J., & Gómez-Carrillo, A. (2019). Agency, embodiment, and enactment in psychosomatic theory and practice. *Medical Humanities*, *45*(2), 169–182. https://doi.org/10.1136/medhum-2018-011618

Kitayama, S., & Markus, H. R. (1994). *Emotion and culture: Empirical studies of mutual influence*. American Psychological Association. https://doi.org/10.1037/10152-000

Kite, J., Huang, B. H., Laird, Y., Grunseit, A., McGill, B., Williams, K., Bellew, B., & Thomas, M. (2022). Influence and effects of weight stigmatisation in media: A systematic review. *eClinical Medicine*, *48*, 101464. https://doi.org/10.1016/j.eclinm.2022.101464

Klasen, H. (2000). A name, what's in a name? The medicalization of hyperactivity, revisited. *Harvard Review of Psychiatry*, *7*(6), 334–344. https://doi.org/10.3109/hrp.7.6.334

Kleinman, A. (1977). Depression, somatization and the new cross-cultural psychiatry. *Social Science and Medicine*, *11*, 3–10.

Kleinman, A. (1987). Anthropology and psychiatry: The role of culture in cross-cultural research on illness. *British Journal of Psychiatry*, *151*, 447–454. https://doi.org/10.1192/bjp.151.4.447

Klier, K., Rommerskirchen, T., & Brixius, K. (2022). #fitspiration: A comparison of the sport-related social media usage and its impact on body image in young adults. *BMC Psychology*, *10*, 320. https://doi.org/10.1186/s40359-022-01027-9

Kneeland, J. (2023). *Body neutral: A revolutionary guide to overcoming body image issues*. Penguin Books.

Kohn, L. A. (1963). Charles Darwin's chronic ill health. *Bulletin of the History of Medicine*, *37*(3), 239–256.

Kosic, A., Lindholm, P., Järvholm, K., Hedman-Lagerlöf, E., & Axelsson, E. (2020). Three decades of increase in health anxiety: Systematic review and meta-analysis of birth cohort changes in university student samples from 1985 to 2017. *Journal of Anxiety Disorders*, *71*, 102208. https://doi.org/10.1016/j.janxdis.2020.102208

Köteles, F., Simor, P., Czető, M., Sárog, N., & Szemerszky, R. (2016). Modern health worries – the dark side of spirituality? *Scandinavian Journal of Psychology*, *57*(4), 313–320. https://doi.org/10.1111/sjop.12297

Köteles, F., Szemerszky, R., Petrie, K., & Nordin, S. (2023). Modern health worries and annoyance from environmental factors are largely unrelated to smoking, alcohol consumption, and physical activity. *Journal of Psychosomatic Research*, *172*, 111417. https://doi.org/10.1016/j.jpsychores.2023.111417

Kőváry, Z. (2024). A history of existential psychology. In *Introduction to existential psychology* (Vol. 1). Routledge. https://doi.org/10.4324/9781032703107

Kraaijeveld, S. R., & Jamrozik, E. (2022). Moralization and mismoralization in public health. *Medicine, Health Care and Philosophy*, *25*(4), 655–669. https://doi.org/10.1007/s11019-022-10103-1

Krämer, A., & Winkler, P. (2024). Overcoming the "blame game" in strategic climate communication: From decoupling accusations toward an arena-spanning agenda. *Journal of Communication Management*, *28*(1), 41–57. https://doi.org/10.1108/JCOM-12-2022-0132

Kresovich, A., Reffner Collins, M. K., Riffe, D., & Carpentier, F. R. D. (2021). A content analysis of mental health discourse in popular rap music. *JAMA Pediatrics*, *175*(3), 286–292. https://doi.org/10.1001/jamapediatrics.2020.5155

Kristensen, D. B., & Prigge, C. (2018). Human/technology associations in self-tracking practices. In B. Ajana (Ed.), *Self-Tracking: Empirical and Philosophical Investigations* (pp. 43–61). Palgrave Macmillan.

Krys, K., de Almeida, I., Wasiel, A., & Vignoles, V. L. (2024a). WEIRD-Confucian comparisons: Ongoing cultural biases in psychology's evidence base and some recommendations for improving global representation. *American Psychologist*. https://doi.org/10.1037/amp0001298

Krys, K., Kostoula, O., van Tilburg, W. A. P., Mosca, O., Lee, J. H., Maricchiolo, F., Kosiarczyk, A., Kocimska-Bortnowska, A., Torres, C., Hitokoto, H., Liew, K., Bond, M. H., Lun, V. M., Vignoles, V. L., Zelenski, J. M., Haas, B. W., Park, J., Vauclair, C. M., Kwiatkowska, A., . . . Uchida, Y. (2024b). Happiness maximization is a WEIRD way of living. *Perspectives on Psychological Science*. Advance online publication. https://doi.org/10.1177/17456916231208367

Kwok, R. H. M. (1968). Chinese-restaurant syndrome. *New England Journal of Medicine*, *278*(14), 796. https://doi.org/10.1056/NEJM196804042781403

Kwon, D. (2023, September 1). What is narcissism? Science confronts a widely misunderstood phenomenon: Researchers debate whether grandiosity always masks vulnerability. *Scientific American*. https://www.scientificamerican.com/article/what-is-narcissism-science-confronts-a-widely-misunderstood-phenomenon1/

Lack, C. W., & Rousseau, J. (2022). Mental health, pop psychology, and the misunderstanding of clinical psychology. In *Reference module in neuroscience and biobehavioral psychology*. https://doi.org/10.1016/B978-0-12-818697-8.00052-2

Ladwig, G., Tanck, J. A., Quittkat, H. L., & Vocks, S. (2024). Risks and benefits of social media trends: The influence of "fitspiration," "body positivity," and text-based "body neutrality" on body dissatisfaction and affect in women with and without eating disorders. *Body Image, 50,* 101749. https://doi.org/10.1016/j.bodyim.2024.101749

Ladyka, D., Kumar, M. M., & Docter, A. D. (2023). A brief history of fad diets and diet culture. In M. M. Kumar & A. Dixon Docter (Eds.), *Fad diets and adolescents*. Springer. https://doi.org/10.1007/978-3-031-10565-4_2

Lagan, S., Aquino, P., Emerson, M. R., Fortuna, K., Walker, R., & Torous, J. (2020). Actionable health app evaluation: Translating expert frameworks into objective metrics. *npj Digital Medicine*, *3*, 100. https://doi.org/10.1038/s41746-020-00312-9

Lahey, B. B., Tiemeier, H., & Krueger, R. F. (2022). Seven reasons why binary diagnostic categories should be replaced with empirically sounder and less stigmatizing dimensions. *JCPP Advances*, *2*(4), e12108. https://doi.org/10.1002/jcv2.12108

Lakin, K., & Kane, S. (2022). Peoples' expectations of healthcare: A conceptual review and proposed analytical framework. *Social Science & Medicine*, *292*, 114636. https://doi.org/10.1016/j.socscimed.2021.114636

Lamarche, L., Bailey, K. A., Awan, A., Risdon, C., Pauw, G., & Vinoski Thomas, E. (2020). Exploring primary care providers' understandings of body image in patient care. *Body Image, 35,* 161–170. https://doi.org/10.1016/j.bodyim.2020.09.001

Lane, P. (2024a). *Understanding and coping with illness anxiety*. Routledge.

Lane, P. (2024b, September 19). How wearable technology can worsen health anxiety. *Psychology Today*. https://www.psychologytoday.com/us/blog/am-i-dying/202409/how-wearable-technology-can-worsen-health-anxiety

Lasch, C. (1979). *The culture of narcissism: American life in an age of diminishing expectations*. Norton.

Latour, B. (2005). *Reassembling the social: An introduction to actor-network-theory*. Oxford University Press.
Lau, C. K. Y., Saad, A., Camara, B., Rahman, D., & Bolea-Alamanac, B. (2024). Acceptability of digital mental health interventions for depression and anxiety: Systematic review. *Journal of Medical Internet Research, 26*, e52609. https://doi.org/10.2196/52609
Lebel, S., Mutsaers, B., Tomei, C., Leclair, C. S., Jones, G., Petricone-Westwood, D., Rutkowski, N., Ta, V., Trudel, G., Laflamme, S. Z., Lavigne, A. A., & Dinkel, A. (2020). Health anxiety and illness-related fears across diverse chronic illnesses: A systematic review on conceptualization, measurement, prevalence, course, and correlates. *PLoS ONE, 15*(7), e0234124. https://doi.org/10.1371/journal.pone.0234124
Lebwohl, B., & Leffler, D. A. (2015). Exploring the strange new world of non-celiac gluten sensitivity. *Clinical Gastroenterology and Hepatology, 13*(9), 1613–1614. https://doi.org/10.1016/j.cgh.2015.07.023
Léger-Goodes, T., Malboeuf-Hurtubise, C., Mastine, T., Généreux, M., Paradis, P. O., & Camden, C. (2022). Eco-anxiety in children: A scoping review of the mental health impacts of the awareness of climate change. *Frontiers in Psychology, 13*, 872544. https://doi.org/10.3389/fpsyg.2022.872544
LeMesurier, J. L. (2017). Uptaking race: Genre, MSG, and Chinese dinner. *Poroi, 12*(2), 7. https://doi.org/10.13008/2151-2957.1253
Lerner, J. S., & Keltner, D. (2000). Beyond valence: Toward a model of emotion-specific influences on judgement and choice. *Cognition and Emotion, 14*(4), 473–493. https://doi.org/10.1080/026999300402763
Lerner, M. J. (1970). The desire for justice and reactions to victims. In J. Macaulay & L. Berkowitz (Eds.), *Altruism and helping behavior* (pp. 205–229). Academic Press.
Lerner, M. J. (1980). *The belief in a just world: A fundamental delusion*. Plenum Press.
Levinovitz, A. (2015). *The gluten lie and other myths about what you eat*. Regan Arts.
Lewis, T. (2006). Seeking health information on the internet: Lifestyle choice or bad attack of cyberchondria? *Media, Culture & Society, 28*(4), 521–539. https://doi.org/10.1177/0163443706065027
Lewis-Fernández, R., & Kleinman, A. (1994). Culture, personality, and psychopathology. *Journal of Abnormal Psychology, 103*(1), 67–71. https://doi.org/10.1037/0021-843X.103.1.67
Leykin, Y., Muñoz, R. F., & Contreras, O. (2012). Are consumers of internet health information "cyberchondriacs"? Characteristics of 24,965 users of a depression screening site. *Depression and Anxiety, 29*(1), 71–77. https://doi.org/10.1002/da.20848
Li, J., Ma, W., Zhang, M., Wang, P., Liu, Y., & Ma, S. (2021). Know yourself: Physical and psychological self-awareness with lifelog. *Frontiers in Digital Health, 3*, 676824. https://doi.org/10.3389/fdgth.2021.676824
Lim, T., Dwirischcka, F., & Chandraputri, A. (2023, November 13). Inside culture: Understanding the dark side of self-care among Asian youth. *WARC*. https://www.warc.com/newsandopinion/opinion/inside-culture-understanding-the-dark-side-of-self-care-among-asian-youth/en-gb/6422
Lim, W. M. (2016). Understanding the selfie phenomenon: Current insights and future research directions. *European Journal of Marketing, 50*(9–10), 1773–1788. https://doi.org/10.1108/EJM-07-2015-0484
Limpanopparat, S., Gibson, E., & Harris, A. (2024). User engagement, attitudes, and the effectiveness of chatbots as a mental health intervention: A systematic review. *Computers in Human Behavior: Artificial Humans, 2*, 100081. https://doi.org/10.1016/j.chbah.2024.100081
Linardon, J., McClure, Z., Tylka, T. L., & Fuller-Tyszkiewicz, M. (2022). Body appreciation and its psychological correlates: A systematic review and meta-analysis. *Body Image, 42*, 287–296. https://doi.org/10.1016/j.bodyim.2022.07.003

Liu, S., Yang, H., Cheng, M., & Miao, T. (2022). Family dysfunction and cyberchondria among Chinese adolescents: A moderated mediation model. *International Journal of Environmental Research and Public Health, 19*(15), 9716. https://doi.org/10.3390/ijerph19159716

Livneh, H. (2019). The use of generic avoidant coping scales for psychosocial adaptation to chronic illness and disability: A systematic review. *Health Psychology Open, 6*(2), 2055102919891396. https://doi.org/10.1177/2055102919891396

Lock, S. (2022, October 28). Disney introduces first plus-size heroine in animated short *Reflect. The Guardian.* https://www.theguardian.com/film/2022/oct/28/disney-reflect-plus-sized-heroine

Lomas, T., Waters, L., Williams, P., Oades, L. G., & Kern, M. L. (2021). Third wave positive psychology: Broadening towards complexity. *The Journal of Positive Psychology, 16*(5), 660–674. https://doi.org/10.1080/17439760.2020.1805501

Lomborg, S., & Frandsen, K. (2016). Self-tracking as communication. *Information, Communication & Society, 19*(7), 1015–1027. https://doi.org/10.1080/1369118X.2015.1067710

López-Gil, J. F., Tárraga-López, P. J., Hershey, M. S., López-Bueno, R., Gutiérrez-Espinoza, H., Soler-Marín, A., Fernández-Montero, A., & Victoria-Montesinos, D. (2023). Overall proportion of orthorexia nervosa symptoms: A systematic review and meta-analysis including 30,476 individuals from 18 countries. *Journal of Global Health, 13*, 04087. https://doi.org/10.7189/jogh.13.04087

Lorde, A. (n.d.). Breaking isolation: Self-care and community care tools for our people. *The Audre Lorde Project.* https://alp.org/breaking-isolation-self-care-and-community-care-tools-our-people

Luhmann, N. (1993). *Risk: A sociological theory*. Walter de Gruyter.

Lupton, D. (1993). Risk as moral danger: The social and political functions of risk discourse in public health. *International Journal of Health Services, 23*(3), 425–435. https://doi.org/10.2190/16AY-E2GC-DFLD-51X2

Lupton, D. (1994). Toward the development of critical health communication praxis. *Health Communication, 6*(1), 55–67. https://doi.org/10.1207/s15327027hc0601_4

Lupton, D. (2012). M-health and health promotion: The digital cyborg and surveillance society. *Social Theory & Health, 10*(3), 229–244. https://doi.org/10.1057/sth.2012.6

Lupton, D. (2013). The digitally engaged patient: Self-monitoring and self-care in the digital health era. *Social Theory & Health, 11*, 256–270. https://doi.org/10.1057/sth.2013.10

Lupton, D. (2014). Critical perspectives on digital health technologies. *Sociology Compass, 8*(12), 1344–1359. https://doi.org/10.1111/soc4.12226

Lupton, D. (2016). *The quantified self: A sociology of self-tracking*. Polity Press.

Lupton, D. (2018). *Digital health: Critical and cross-disciplinary perspectives*. Routledge.

Lupton, D. (2023). *Risk* (3rd ed.) Routledge.

Luthar, S. S., Cicchetti, D., & Becker, B. (2000). The construct of resilience: A critical evaluation and guidelines for future work. *Child Development, 71*(3), 543–562. https://doi.org/10.1111/1467-8624.00164

Lyons, A. C., & Forde, E. M. (2004). Food allergy in young adults: Perceptions and psychological effects. *Journal of Health Psychology, 9*(4), 497–504. https://doi.org/10.1177/1359105304044032

Lyons, R.D. (1968, May 19). 'Chinese restaurant syndrome' puzzles doctors. *The New York Times*. https://www.nytimes.com/1968/05/19/archives/-chinese-restaurant-syndrome-puzzles-doctors.html

Lythe, K. E., Moll, J., Gethin, J. A., Workman, C. I., Green, S., Lambon Ralph, M. A., Deakin, J. F., & Zahn, R. (2015). Self-blame-selective hyperconnectivity between anterior temporal and subgenual cortices and prediction of recurrent depressive episodes. *JAMA Psychiatry, 72*(11), 1119–1126. https://doi.org/10.1001/jamapsychiatry.2015.1813

Ma, Y., & Kroemer, G. (2024). The cancer-immune dialogue in the context of stress. *Nature Reviews Immunology*, *24*(4), 264–281. https://doi.org/10.1038/s41577-023-00949-8

MacNeill, A. L., Doucet, S., & Luke, A. (2024). Effectiveness of a mental health chatbot for people with chronic diseases: Randomized controlled trial. *JMIR Formative Research*, *8*, e50025. https://doi.org/10.2196/50025

Macrynikola, N., Mir, Z., Gopal, T., Rodriguez, E., Li, S., Cox, M., Yeh, G., & Torous, J. (2024). The impact of mindfulness apps on psychological processes of change: A systematic review. *npj Mental Health Research*, *3*, 14. https://doi.org/10.1038/s44184-023-00048-5

Madanian, S., Nakarada-Kordic, I., Reay, S., & Chetty, T. (2023). Patients' perspectives on digital health tools. *PEC Innovation*, *2*, 100171. https://doi.org/10.1016/j.pecinn.2023.100171

Maes, C., Trekels, J., Tylka, T. L., & Vandenbosch, L. (2021). The positive body image among adolescents scale (PBIAS): Development and validation of a new measure. *Body Image*, *39*, 63–75. https://doi.org/10.1016/j.bodyim.2021.05.006

Maftei, A., & Holman, A. C. (2020). Cyberchondria during the coronavirus pandemic: The effects of neuroticism and optimism. *Frontiers in Psychology*, *11*, 567345. https://doi.org/10.3389/fpsyg.2020.567345

Magkos, F., Tetens, I., Bügel, S. G., Felby, C., Schacht, S. R., Hill, J. O., Ravussin, E., & Astrup, A. (2020). The environmental foodprint of obesity. *Obesity*, *28*(1), 73–79. https://doi.org/10.1002/oby.22657

Magnusson, J. (Director). (2020). *Maddy, the model* [Film]. B-Reel Films.

Mahdi, G. S. (2006). The Atkins diet controversy. *Annals of Saudi Medicine*, *26*(3), 244–245. https://doi.org/10.5144/0256-4947.2006.244

Mahdiani, H., & Ungar, M. (2021). The dark side of resilience. *Adversity and Resilience Science*, *2*(2), 147–155. https://doi.org/10.1007/s42844-021-00031-z

Makris, G., Papageorgiou, N., Panagopoulos, D., & Glatz Brubakk, K. (2021). A diagnostic challenge in an unresponsive refugee child improving with neurosurgery – a case report. *Oxford Medical Case Reports*, *2021*(5), omab020. https://doi.org/10.1093/omcr/omab020

Malla, A., & Gold, I. (2024). Public discourse on mental health: A critical view. *Journal of Psychiatry and Neuroscience*, *49*(2), E126–E131. https://doi.org/10.1503/jpn.230161

Mani, M., Kavanagh, D. J., Hides, L., & Stoyanov, S. R. (2015). Review and evaluation of mindfulness-based iPhone apps. *JMIR mHealth and uHealth*, *3*(3), e82. https://doi.org/10.2196/mhealth.4328

Mansharamani, V. (2015, May 5). We're in a gluten-free bubble that is about to burst. *Fortune*. https://fortune.com/2015/05/05/gluten-free-foods/

Mantler, J., Schellenberg, E. G., & Page, J. S. (2003). Attributions for serious illness: Are controllability, responsibility, and blame different constructs? *Canadian Journal of Behavioural Science/Revue canadienne des sciences du comportement*, *35*(2), 142–152. https://doi.org/10.1037/h0087196

Maon, S., Hassan, N. M., & Seman, S. A. A. (2017). Online health information seeking behavior pattern. *Journal of Computational and Theoretical Nanoscience*, *23*, 10582–10585. https://doi.org/10.1166/asl.2017.10107

Markoff, J. (2008, November 24). Microsoft examines the causes of cyberchondria. *The New York Times*. https://www.nytimes.com/2008/11/25/technology/internet/25symptoms.html

Markula, P., Burns, M., & Riley, S. (2008). Introducing critical bodies: Representations, identities and practices of weight and body management. In S. Riley, M. Burns, H. Frith, S. Wiggins, & P. Markula (Eds.), *Critical bodies* (pp. 1–21). Palgrave Macmillan.

Martin, M. W. (2001). Responsibility for health and blaming victims. *Journal of Medical Humanities*, *22*(2), 95–114. https://doi.org/10.1023/A:1009074811781

Marziliano, A., Moyer, A., & Tuman, M. (2024). Posttraumatic growth in the context of illness. In R. Berger (Ed.), *The Routledge international handbook of posttraumatic growth*. https://doi.org/10.4324/9781032208688

Massey, A. (2019, June 24). Medicalising everyday life doesn't help anyone's mental health. *The Guardian*. https://www.theguardian.com/commentisfree/2019/jun/24/medicalising-mental-health-ilnness-nhs

Maurer, M. M. (2024). Suggested metatheory for positive psychology: The organismic systems theory. *International Journal of Wellbeing, 14*(3). https://doi.org/10.5502/ijw.v14i3.2547

May, M. (2024). How virtual reality therapy is shaping mental health. *Nature Medicine, 30*(7), 1797–1799. https://doi.org/10.1038/d41591-024-00032-2

May, R. (2015). *The meaning of anxiety*. W. W. Norton & Co. (Original work published 1977)

Mazidi, M., Kami, M., & Macleod, C. (2024). Illuminating the association between intolerance of uncertainty and health anxiety: The mediating role of worry. *Journal of Emotion and Psychopathology*. https://doi.org/10.13140/RG.2.2.22048.10243

Mazurkiewicz, N., Krefta, J., & Lipowska, M. (2021). Attitudes towards appearance and body-related stigma among young women with obesity and psoriasis. *Frontiers in Psychiatry, 12*. https://doi.org/10.3389/fpsyt.2021.788439

McDougall, J. (1989). *Theaters of the body: A psychoanalytic approach to psychosomatic illness*. W. W. Norton & Company.

McElroy, E., & Shevlin, M. (2014). The development and initial validation of the cyberchondria severity scale (CSS). *Journal of Anxiety Disorders, 28*(2), 259–265. https://doi.org/10.1016/j.janxdis.2013.12.007

McEvoy, P. M., Carleton, R. N., Correa, K., Shankman, S. A., & Shihata, S. (2019). Intolerance of uncertainty. In B. O. Olatunji (Ed.), *The Cambridge handbook of anxiety and related disorders* (pp. 196–226). Cambridge University Press. https://doi.org/10.1017/9781108140416.008

McGuire, B. (2020). Buddhist-inspired self-tracking apps: Tracking emotions and values in a digital era. *Journal of the Japanese Association for Digital Humanities, 5*(2), 43–60. https://doi.org/10.17928/jjadh.5.2_43

McIntyre, R. S., Ismail, Z., Watling, C. P., Weiss, C., Meehan, S. R., Musingarimi, P., & Thase, M. E. (2022). Patient-reported outcome measures for life engagement in mental health: A systematic review. *Journal of Patient-Reported Outcomes, 6*(1), 62. https://doi.org/10.1186/s41687-022-00468-5

McKinney, S. M., Sieniek, M., Godbole, V., Godwin, J., Antropova, N., Ashrafian, H., Back, T., Chesus, M., Corrado, G. S., Darzi, A., Etemadi, M., Garcia-Vicente, F., Gilbert, F. J., Halling-Brown, M., Hassabis, D., Jansen, S., Karthikesalingam, A., Kelly, C. J., King, D., . . . Shetty, S. (2020). International evaluation of an AI system for breast cancer screening. *Nature, 577*(7788), 89–94. https://doi.org/10.1038/s41586-019-1799-6

McManus, F., Leung, C., Muse, K., & Williams, J. M. G. (2015). Understanding 'cyberchondria': An interpretive phenomenological analysis of the purpose, methods and impact of seeking health information online for those with health anxiety. *The Cognitive Behaviour Therapist, 7*, e21.

McWhorter, K. L. (2020). Obesity acceptance: Body positivity and clinical risk factors. In D. C. Gaze & A. Kibel (Eds.), *Cardiac diseases – novel aspects of cardiac risk, cardiorenal pathology and cardiac interventions*. IntechOpen. https://doi.org/10.5772/intechopen.93540

Medaris, A. (2024). How to harness the power of therapy-speak. *APA Monitor on Psychology, 55*(6). https://www.apa.org/monitor/2024/09/therapy-speak

Medical Director. (2019, May 27). Health anxiety, Doctor Google, and a generation of 'worried well'. *Clinical Practice*. https://www.medicaldirector.com/news/clinical-practice/2019/05/health-anxiety-doctor-google-and-a-generation-of-worried-well

Meerholz, E. W., Spears, R., & Epstude, K. (2019). Having pity on our victims to save ourselves: Compassion reduces self-critical emotions and self-blame about past harmful behavior among those who highly identify with their past self. *PLoS ONE, 14*(12), e0223945. https://doi.org/10.1371/journal.pone.0223945

Meland, E., Haugland, S., & Breidablik, H. J. (2007). Body image and perceived health in adolescence. *Health Education Research*, *22*(3), 342–350. https://doi.org/10.1093/her/cyl085

Mento, C., Damiani, F., La Versa, M., Cedro, C., Muscatello, M. R. A., Bruno, A., Fabio, R. A., & Silvestri, M. C. (2023). Eco-anxiety: An evolutionary line from psychology to psychopathology. *Medicina*, *59*(12), 2053. https://doi.org/10.3390/medicina59122053

Menzel, J. E., & Levine, M. P. (2011). Embodying experiences and the promotion of positive body image: The example of competitive athletics. In R. M. Calogero, S. Tantleff-Dunn, & J. K. Thompson (Eds.), *Self-objectification in women: Causes, consequences, and counteractions* (pp. 163–186). American Psychological Association.

Merino, M., Tornero-Aguilera, J. F., Rubio-Zarapuz, A., Villanueva-Tobaldo, C. V., Martín-Rodríguez, A., & Clemente-Suárez, V. J. (2024). Body perceptions and psychological well-being: A review of the impact of social media and physical measurements on self-esteem and mental health with a focus on body image satisfaction and its relationship with cultural and gender factors. *Healthcare*, *12*(14), 1396. https://doi.org/10.3390/healthcare12141396

Merriam-Webster Dictionary. (n.d.). MSG symptom complex. *Merriam-Webster.com Dictionary*. https://www.merriam-webster.com/dictionary/MSG%20symptom%20complex

Meskó, B. (2020). Digital health technologies and well-being in the future. *IT Professional*, *22*(1), 0–23. https://doi.org/10.1109/MITP.2019.2963121

Meskó, B. (2023, October 19). Digital health anxiety: When wellness tech becomes a stressor. *The Medical Futurist*. https://medicalfuturist.com/digital-health-anxiety-when-wellness-tech-becomes-a-stressor

Meskó, B., Drobni, Z., Bényei, É., Gergely, B., & Győrffy, Z. (2017). Digital health is a cultural transformation of traditional healthcare. *mHealth*, *3*, 38. https://doi.org/10.21037/mhealth.2017.08.07

Mestre-Bach, G., & Potenza, M. N. (2023). Cyberchondria: A growing concern during the COVID-19 pandemic and a possible addictive disorder? *Current Addiction Reports*, *10*(1), 77–96. https://doi.org/10.1007/s40429-022-00462-3

Meštrović, S. G. (1997). *Postemotional society*. Sage Publications.

Metcalfe, D. D., Sampson, H. A., & Simon, R. A. (2013). *Food allergy: Adverse reactions to foods and food additives*. Blackwell Publishing.

Meyers, B. C. (2023). *I am more than my body: The body neutral journey*. G.P. Putnam's Sons.

Mihelj, S., Kondor, K., & Štětka, V. (2022). Establishing trust in experts during a crisis: Expert trustworthiness and media use during the COVID-19 pandemic. *Science Communication*, *44*(3), 292–319. https://doi.org/10.1177/10755470221100558

Milbury, K., Badr, H., & Carmack, C. L. (2012). The role of blame in the psychosocial adjustment of couples coping with lung cancer. *Annals of Behavioral Medicine*, *44*(3), 331–340. https://doi.org/10.1007/s12160-012-9402-5

Milton, A., Hambleton, A., Roberts, A., Davenport, T., Flego, A., Burns, J., & Hickie, I. (2021). Body image distress and its associations from an international sample of men and women across the adult life span: Web-based survey study. *JMIR Formative Research*, *5*(11), e25329. https://doi.org/10.2196/25329

Min, A. D. (2021, April 21). Don't Covid-shame. *The Harvard Crimson*. https://www.thecrimson.com/article/2021/4/21/min-dont-covid-shame/

Moench, M. (2023, November 22). New data shows a global surge in searches related to 'climate anxiety.' *Time*. https://time.com/6338759/climate-change-anxiety-google-search-trend/

Mohamed, F., Mamede, S., Mohamedani, M., Al Alwan, I., Magzoub, M. E. M., & Schmidt, H. G. (2016). The effect of patients' appearance on doctors' diagnostic decision making: Do poor people get poorer medical care? *Health Professions Education*, *2*(1), 4. https://doi.org/10.1016/j.hpe.2016.01.011

Mohammadinia, N., Nasehi, A., & Niusha, B. (2024). The effect of health literacy on health anxiety with the mediation of cyberchondria and cognitive flexibility in breast cancer patients. *Iranian Journal of Psychiatry and Nursing, 11*(6), 129–140. http://ijpn.ir/article-1–2273-en.html

Monaghan, L. F., Rich, E., & Bombak, A. E. (2022). *Rethinking obesity: Critical perspectives in crisis times*. Routledge.

Montgomery, S. (2010). The rise of the body positive movement. *Sharnanigans.com*. http://www.sharnanigans.com/2010/12/the-rise-of-thebody-positive-movement/

Morris, A. (2019). *The politics of weight: Feminist dichotomies of power in dieting*. Palgrave Macmillan. https://doi.org/10.1007/978-3-030-13670-3_5

Morrison, S. A. (2022). Moving in a hotter world: Maintaining adequate childhood fitness as a climate change countermeasure. *Temperature, 10*(2), 179–197.

Morselli, P., & Grattini, S. (1970). Monosodium glutamate and the Chinese restaurant syndrome. *Nature, 227*, 611–612. https://doi.org/10.1038/227611a0

Mosby, I. (2009). 'That won-ton soup headache': The Chinese restaurant syndrome, MSG and the making of American food, 1968–1980. *Social History of Medicine, 22*(1), 133–151. https://doi.org/10.1093/shm/hkn098

Moussaoui, L. S., Claxton, N., & Desrichard, O. (2021). Fear appeals to promote better health behaviors: An investigation of potential mediators. *Health Psychology and Behavioral Medicine, 9*(1), 600–618. https://doi.org/10.1080/21642850.2021.1947290

Murray, S. (2008). Pathologizing 'fatness': Medical authority and popular culture. *Sociology of Sport Journal, 25*, 7–21. https://doi.org/10.1123/ssj.25.1.7

Mushtaq, R., Shoib, S., Shah, T., & Mushtaq, S. (2014). Relationship between loneliness, psychiatric disorders and physical health: A review on the psychological aspects of loneliness. *Journal of Clinical and Diagnostic Research, 8*(9), WE01–WE04. https://doi.org/10.7860/JCDR/2014/10077.4828

Muttarak, R. (2018). Normalization of plus size and the danger of unseen overweight and obesity in England. *Obesity, 26*(7), 1125–1129. https://doi.org/10.1002/oby.22204

Mythen, G. (2021). The critical theory of world risk society: A retrospective analysis. *Risk Analysis, 41*(3), 533–543. https://doi.org/10.1111/risa

Nagler, R. H., Vogel, R. I., Rothman, A. J., Yzer, M. C., & Gollust, S. E. (2023). Vulnerability to the effects of conflicting health information: Testing the moderating roles of trust in news media and research literacy. *Health Education & Behavior, 50*(2), 224–233. https://doi.org/10.1177/10901981221110833

Nakayachi, K. (2013). The unintended effects of risk-refuting information on anxiety. *Risk Analysis, 33*(1), 80–91. https://doi.org/10.1111/j.1539-6924.2012.01852.x

Nasiri, M., Mohammadkhani, S., Akbari, M., & Alilou, M. M. (2023). The structural model of cyberchondria based on personality traits, health-related metacognition, cognitive bias, and emotion dysregulation. *Frontiers in Psychiatry, 13*, 960055. https://doi.org/10.3389/fpsyt.2022.960055

Natividad, N. (2022, October 10). What to do if you can't afford therapy. *Vice*. https://www.vice.com/en/article/therapy-mental-health-wellbeing-meditation

Neff, K. D. (2003). Self-compassion: An alternative conceptualization of a healthy attitude toward oneself. *Self and Identity, 2*(2), 85–101. https://doi.org/10.1080/15298860309032

Nehring, D., Madsen, O. J., Cabanas, E., Mills, C., & Kerrigan, D. (Eds.). (2020). *Routledge international handbook of global therapeutic cultures*. Routledge.

Ngenye, L., & Wright, K. (2022). Online social support groups/communities: Implications of theoretical and empirical findings for individuals coping with health concerns. In *Research anthology on improving health literacy through patient communication and mass media* (Chapter 20). IGI Global. https://doi.org/10.4018/978-1-6684-2414-8.ch020

Nickel, P. J., Loosman, I., Frank, L., & Vinnikova, A. (2023). Justice and empowerment through digital health: Ethical challenges and opportunities. *Digital Society*, *2*, 42. https://doi.org/10.1007/s44206-023-00075-x

Nickel, P. J., Loosman, I., Frank, L., & Vinnikova, A. (2024). Digital health empowerment, autonomy, and the capability approach: Reply to de Proost and Grey. *DISO*, *3*, 32. https://doi.org/10.1007/s44206-024-00120-3

Niedzwiedz, C., & Katikireddi, S. V. (2023). Determinants of eco-anxiety: Cross-national study of 52,219 participants from 25 European countries. *European Journal of Public Health*, *33*(Suppl 2), ckad160.069. https://doi.org/10.1093/eurpub/ckad160.069

Niemeyer, H., & Knaevelsrud, C. (2023). Socioeconomic status and access to psychotherapy. *Journal of Clinical Psychology*, *79*(4), 937–953. https://doi.org/10.1002/jclp.23449

Nierenberg, A. (2020, January 16). The campaign to redefine 'Chinese restaurant syndrome'. *The New York Times*. https://www.nytimes.com/2020/01/16/dining/msg-chinese-restaurant-syndrome-merriam-webster-dictionary.html

Nieslanik, T. (2024, October 4). Wearable fitness trackers are making us anxious – here's how to stop it. *National Geographic*. https://www.nationalgeographic.com/science/article/how-wearable-tech-can-trigger-anxiety-and-how-to-manage-it

Nietzsche, F. (2009). *Ecce homo: How one becomes what one is* (W. Kaufmann, Trans.). Oxford University Press. (Original work published 1888)

Nightingale, J., & Cromby, J. (2001). Critical psychology and the ideology of individualism. *Journal of Critical Psychology, Counselling and Psychotherapy*, *1*(2), 117–128. https://www.researchgate.net/publication/228490083_Critical_psychology_and_the_ideology_of_individualism

Niland, B., & Cash, B. D. (2018). Health benefits and adverse effects of a gluten-free diet in non-celiac disease patients. *Gastroenterology & Hepatology*, *14*(2), 82–91. https://www.ncbi.nlm.nih.gov/pmc/articles/PMC5866307/

Non, A. L., Román, J. C., Clausing, E. S., Gilman, S. E., Loucks, E. B., Buka, S. L., Appleton, A. A., & Kubzansky, L. D. (2020). Optimism and social support predict healthier adult behaviors despite socially disadvantaged childhoods. *International Journal of Behavioral Medicine*, *27*(2), 200–212. https://doi.org/10.1007/s12529-020-09849-w

Nopper, T. K., & Zelickson, E. (2023, June 21). Wellness capitalism: Employee health, the benefits maze, and worker control. *Data & Society*. https://datasociety.net/library/wellness-capitalism-employee-health-the-benefits-maze-and-worker-control/

Northup, T., & Liebler, C. M. (2010). The good, the bad, and the beautiful: Beauty ideals on the Disney and Nickelodeon channels. *Journal of Children and Media*, *4*(3), 265–282. https://doi.org/10.1080/17482798.2010.496917

Norwood, F. B. (2021). Perceived impact of information signals on opinions about gluten-free diets. *PLoS ONE*, *16*(4), e0248570. https://doi.org/10.1371/journal.pone.0248570

Nucci, J. (2025). *Psychobabble: Viral mental health myths & the truths to set you free*. HarperOne.

Oishi, S., & Westgate, E. C. (2022). A psychologically rich life: Beyond happiness and meaning. *Psychological Review*, *129*(4), 790–811. https://doi.org/10.1037/rev0000317

Oliver, M. D. D., Baldwin, D. R., & Datta, S. (2018). Health to wellness: A review of wellness models and transitioning back to health. *The International Journal of Health, Wellness, and Society*, *9*(1), 41–56. https://doi.org/10.18848/2156-8960/CGP/v09i01/41-56

Omelichkin, O. V. (2020). The principles and rules of bioethics. *Bulletin of Social Sciences and Humanities*, *1*(2), 41–47. (In Russian)

Oostrum, J. M. van. (2024). *Exploring the impact of wearable devices on perceived stress and health anxiety: A mixed-methods approach* (Student thesis). University of Twente.

Orbach, S. (2010). *Bodies*. Profile Books.

O'Riordan, T., Marris, C., & Langford, I. (1997). Images of science underlying public perceptions of risk. In *Science, policy and risk* (pp. 13–30). Royal Society.

Outland, L. (2010). Intuitive eating: A holistic approach to weight control. *Holistic Nursing Practice, 24*(1), 35–43. https://doi.org/10.1097/HNP.0b013e3181c8e560
Oxford Dictionaries. (2015). *Self-tracking*. Oxford Dictionaries.
Pallavi, P., Bakhla, A. K., Kisku, R. R., Guria, R., Mundu, M., & Bala, R. (2022). Excessive and unreliable health information and its predictability for anxiety: A cross-sectional observational study. *Cureus, 14*(11), e31247. https://doi.org/10.7759/cureus.31247
Palmquist, E., Petrie, K. J., & Nordin, S. (2017). Psychometric properties and normative data for a Swedish version of the modern health worries scale. *International Journal of Behavioral Medicine, 24*(1), 54–65. https://doi.org/10.1007/s12529-016-9576-5
Panchuk, M. (2024) What doesn't kill me makes me stronger? Post-traumatic growth and the problem of suffering. *Religious Studies, 60*(3), 428–444. https://doi.org/10.1017/S0034412523000999
Pantzar, M., & Ruckenstein, M. (2017). Living the metrics: Self-tracking and situated objectivity. *Digital Health, 3*. https://doi.org/10.1177/2055207617712590
Panza, G. A., Armstrong, L. E., Taylor, B. A., Puhl, R. M., Livingston, J., & Pescatello, L. S. (2018). Weight bias among exercise and nutrition professionals: A systematic review. *Obesity Reviews, 19*(11), 1492–1503. https://doi.org/10.1111/obr.12743
Parsons, T. (1951). Illness and the role of the physician: A sociological perspective. *American Journal of Orthopsychiatry, 21*(3), 452–460. https://doi.org/10.1111/j.1939-0025.1951.tb00003.x
Pashazadeh Kan, F., Raoofi, S., Rafiei, S., Khani, S., Hosseinifard, H., Tajik, F., Raoofi, N., Ahmadi, S., Aghalou, S., Torabi, F., Dehnad, A., Rezaei, S., Hosseinipalangi, Z., & Ghashghaee, A. (2021). A systematic review of the prevalence of anxiety among the general population during the COVID-19 pandemic. *Journal of Affective Disorders, 293*, 391–398. https://doi.org/10.1016/j.jad.2021.06.073
Paulsen, R. (2024). *Why we worry: A sociological explanation*. Routledge.
Pawlak, J. (2022). "To portray is to meet": The performativity of Lene Marie Fossen's photographic self-portraits. *Pamiętnik Teatralny, 71*(4), 51–68. https://www.ceeol.com/search/article-detail?id=1098497
Pearl, R. L., & Sheynblyum, M. (2025). How weight bias and stigma undermine healthcare access and utilization. *Current Obesity Reports, 14*(11). https://doi.org/10.1007/s13679-025-00605-3
Pellizzer, M. L., & Wade, T. D. (2023). Developing a definition of body neutrality and strategies for an intervention. *Body Image, 46*, 434–442. https://doi.org/10.1016/j.bodyim.2023.07.006
Péloquin, K., Brassard, A., Arpin, V., Sabourin, S., & Wright, J. (2017). Whose fault is it? Blame predicting psychological adjustment and couple satisfaction in couples seeking fertility treatment. *Journal of Psychosomatic Obstetrics & Gynecology, 39*(1), 64–72. https://doi.org/10.1080/0167482X.2017.1289369
Pennington, N., & Dam, L. (2023). Social interaction, support preferences, and the use of wearable health trackers. *Frontiers in Communication, 8*, 1–11. https://doi.org/10.3389/fcomm.2023.1256452
Peretti-Watel, P. (2003). Neutralization theory and the denial of risk: Some evidence from cannabis use among French adolescents. *British Journal of Sociology, 54*(1), 21–42. https://doi.org/10.1080/0007131032000045888
Perlmutter, D. (2016). *The grain brain whole life plan: Boost brain performance, lose weight, and achieve optimal health*. Brown Spark.
Perry, J. (2021). *Trust in public institutions: Trends and implications for economic security*. United Nations, Department of Economic and Social Affairs.
Petrescu-Mag, R. M., Burny, P., Banatean-Dunea, I., & Petrescu, D. C. (2022). How climate change science is reflected in people's minds: A cross-country study on people's perceptions of climate change. *International Journal of Environmental Research and Public Health, 19*(7), 4280. https://doi.org/10.3390/ijerph19074280

Petrescu-Mag, R. M., Petrescu, D. C., Ivan, A., & Tenter, A. (2023). An intergenerational reading of climate change-health concern nexus: A qualitative study of the Millennials' and Gen Z participants' perceptions. *BMC Public Health*, *23*(1), 484. https://doi.org/10.1186/s12889-023-15353-z

Petrie, K. J., Sivertsen, B., Hysing, M., Broadbent, E., Moss-Morris, R., Eriksen, H. R., & Ursin, H. (2001). Thoroughly modern worries: The relationship of worries about modernity to reported symptoms, health, and medical care utilization. *Journal of Psychosomatic Research*, *51*(1), 395–401. https://doi.org/10.1016/s0022-3999(01)00219–7

Petrie, K. J., & Weinman, J. (2017). The PACE trial: It's time to broaden perceptions and move on. *Journal of Health Psychology*, *22*(9), 1198–1200. https://doi.org/10.1177/1359105317703789

Petrovic, P. (2016). Resignation syndrome: Catatonia? Culture-bound? *Frontiers in Behavioral Neuroscience*, *10*, 7. https://doi.org/10.3389/fnbeh.2016.00007

Pham, N. T., Lee, J. J., Pham, N. H., Phan, T. D. Q., Tran, K., Dang, H. B., Teo, I., Malhotra, C., Finkelstein, E. A., & Ozdemir, S. (2021). The prevalence of perceived stigma and self-blame and their associations with depression, emotional well-being and social well-being among advanced cancer patients: Evidence from the APPROACH cross-sectional study in Vietnam. *BMC Palliative Care*, *20*(1), 104. https://doi.org/10.1186/s12904-021-00803-5

Piatkowski, T. M., Neumann, D. L., Seekis, V., & Dunn, M. (2024). Understanding muscularity, physique anxiety, and the experience of body image enhancement among men and women: A mixed-methods study. *Journal of Community & Applied Social Psychology*. Advance online publication. https://doi.org/10.1002/casp.2800

Pidgeon, N., Kasperson, R. E., & Slovic, P. (2003). *The social amplification of risk*. Cambridge University Press.

Pihkala, P. (2021). Eco-anxiety. In C. Krieg Parker & R. Toivanen (Eds.), *Situating sustainability: A handbook of contexts and concepts* (pp. 119–134). Helsinki University Press.

Plaufcan, M. R., Wamboldt, F. S., & Holm, K. E. (2012). Behavioral and characterological self-blame in chronic obstructive pulmonary disease. *Journal of Psychosomatic Research*, *72*(1), 78–83. https://doi.org/10.1016/j.jpsychores.2011.10.004

Plesa, P. (2023). Authenticization: Consuming commodified authenticity to become "authentic" subjects. *Theory & psychology*, *33*(4), 555–576.

Plush Care Content Team. (2024, September 23). How accurate is mental health advice on TikTok? *Plush Care*. https://plushcare.com/blog/tiktok-mental-health/

Polakovská, L., & Řiháček, T. (2022). What is it like to live with medically unexplained physical symptoms? A qualitative meta-summary. *Psychology and Health, 37*(5), 580–596. https://doi.org/10.1080/08870446.2021.1901900. Epub 2021 Apr 19. PMID: 33872098.

Polloni, L., & Muraro, A. (2020). Anxiety and food allergy: A review of the last two decades. *Clinical & Experimental Allergy*, *50*(4), 420–441. https://doi.org/10.1111/cea.13548

Preskey, N. (2021). Cosmopolitan defends plus-size cover after Twitter users criticise magazine for 'promoting obesity'. *The Independent*. https://www.independent.co.uk/life-style/health-and-families/cosmopolitan-plus-size-cover-covid-b1785984.html

Prior, L. (2003). Belief, knowledge, and expertise: The emergence of the lay expert in medical sociology. *Sociology of Health & Illness*, *25*(1), 41–57. https://doi.org/10.1111/1467-9566.00339

Priven, M., Baum, J., Vieira, E., Fung, T., & Herbold, N. (2015). The influence of a factitious free-from food product label on consumer perceptions of healthfulness. *Journal of the Academy of Nutrition and Dietetics*, *115*(11), 1808–1814. https://doi.org/10.1016/j.jand.2015.03.013

Puhl, R. M., Lessard, L. M., Pearl, R. L., Himmelstein, M. S., & Foster, G. D. (2021). International comparisons of weight stigma: Addressing a void in the field. *International Journal of Obesity*, *45*(9), 1976–1985. https://doi.org/10.1038/s41366-021-00860-z

Pytell, T. E. (2015). *Viktor Frankl's search for meaning: An emblematic 20th century life*. Berghahn Books.

Quinn, T. P., Senadeera, M., Jacobs, S., Coghlan, S., & Le, V. (2021). Trust and medical AI: The challenges we face and the expertise needed to overcome them. *Journal of the American Medical Informatics Association*, *28*(4), 890–894. https://doi.org/10.1093/jamia/ocaa268

Quittkat, H. L., Hartmann, A. S., Düsing, R., Buhlmann, U., & Vocks, S. (2019). Body dissatisfaction, importance of appearance, and body appreciation in men and women over the lifespan. *Frontiers in Psychiatry*, *10*, 864. https://doi.org/10.3389/fpsyt.2019.00864

Race, K. (2012). 'Frequent sipping': Bottled water, the will to health and the subject of hydration. *Body & Society*, *18*(3–4), 72–98.

Radó, N., Girasek, E., Békási, S., & Győrffy, Z. (2022). Digital technology access and health-related internet use among people experiencing homelessness in Hungary: Quantitative survey. *Journal of Medical Internet Research*, *24*(10), e38729. https://doi.org/10.2196/38729

Ramage, J. (2005). *Twentieth-century American success rhetoric: How to construct a suitable self*. Southern Illinois University Press.

Ramphul, K. (2022). "Zoom dysmorphia": The rise of a new issue amidst the pandemic. *Acta Biomedica*, *92*(6), e2021348. https://doi.org/10.23750/abm.v92i6.12523

Ramphul, K., & Mejias, S. G. (2018). Is "Snapchat dysmorphia" a real issue? *Cureus*, *10*(3), e2263. https://doi.org/10.7759/cureus.2263

Rasborg, K. (2012). (World) risk society or new rationalities of risk? A critical discussion of Ulrich Beck's theory of reflexive modernity. *Thesis Eleven*, *108*(1), 3–25. https://doi.org/10.1177/0725513611421479

Rask, C. U., Duholm, C. S., Poulsen, C. M., Rimvall, M. K., & Wright, K. D. (2024). Annual research review: Health anxiety in children and adolescents – developmental aspects and cross-generational influences. *Journal of Child Psychology and Psychiatry*, *65*(4), 413–430. https://doi.org/10.1111/jcpp.13912

Rathbone, J. A., Cruwys, T., Jetten, J., Banas, K., Smyth, L., & Murray, K. (2023). How conceptualizing obesity as a disease affects beliefs about weight, and associated weight stigma and clinical decision-making in health care. *British Journal of Health Psychology*, *28*(2), 291–305. https://doi.org/10.1111/bjhp.12625

Ray, S. J. (2020). *A field guide to climate anxiety: How to keep your cool on a warming planet*. University of California Press.

Raziye, S., Izgi, G., & Nihal, B. (2022). Health literacy and cyberchondria levels in healthcare workers and their relationship with body awareness and physical activity. *Medical Bulletin of Haseki*, *60*(4), 351–357. https://doi.org/10.4274/haseki.galenos.2022.8258

Reker, G. T. (2000). Theoretical perspective, dimensions, and measurement of existential meaning. In G. T. Reker & K. Chamberlain (Eds.), *Exploring existential meaning: Optimizing human development across the life span* (pp. 39–58). Sage.

Reker, G. T., & Chamberlain, K. (Eds.). (2000). *Exploring existential meaning: Optimizing human development across the life span*. Sage.

Renahy, E., & Chauvin, P. (2006). Internet uses for health information seeking: A literature review. *Revue d'Épidémiologie et de Santé Publique*, *54*(3), 263–275. https://doi.org/10.1016/s0398-7620(06)76721-9

Research and Markets. (2025, February 24). Mindfulness meditation apps business analysis report 2025: Development of subscription-based and freemium business models sustains market growth – global forecast to 2030. *GlobeNewswire*. https://www.globenewswire.com/news-release/2025/02/24/3031282/28124/en/Mindfulness-Meditation-Apps-Business-Analysis-Report-2025-Development-of-Subscription-Based-and-Freemium-Business-Models-Sustains-Market-Growth-Global-Forecast-to–2030.html

Rettberg, J. W. (2018). Apps as companions: How quantified self apps become our audience and our companions. In B. Ajana (Ed.), *Self-tracking: Empirical and philosophical investigations* (pp. 27–43). Palgrave Macmillan.
Reveley, J. (2016). Neoliberal meditations: How mindfulness training medicalizes education and responsibilizes young people. *Policy Futures in Education, 14*(4), 497–511. https://doi.org/10.1177/1478210316637972
Reynolds, B., & Seeger, M. W. (2005). Crisis and emergency risk communication as an integrative model. *Journal of Health Communication, 10*(1), 43–57. https://doi.org/10.1080/10810730590904571
Riaz, T., Akram, M., Laila, U., Zainab, R., Khalil, M. T., Iftikhar, M., Ozdemir, F. A., Sołowski, G., Altable, M., Sfera, A., Ibrahim, H. K., & Parmar, P. (2023). Causes, risk factors, and medical consequences of obesity. *International Archives of Integrated Medicine, 10*(8), 39–48.
Richards, E. L. (1941). Following the hypochondriacal child for a decade. *Journal of Pediatrics, 18*, 528–537.
Ridgway, B. D. (2017). *Break your self-help addiction: The 5 keys to total personal freedom*. Morgan James Publishing.
Ridolfi, D. R., & Crowther, J. H. (2013). The link between women's body image disturbances and body-focused cancer screening behaviors: A critical review of the literature and a new integrated model for women. *Body Image, 10*(2), 149–162. https://doi.org/10.1016/j.bodyim.2012.11.003
Riessman, F., & Carroll, D. (1995). *Redefining self-help: Policy and practice*. Jossey-Bass.
Riley, S., Evans, A., & Robson, M. (2019). *Postfeminism and health: Critical psychology and media perspectives*. Routledge.
Rimke, H. (2020). Self-help, therapeutic industries, and neoliberalism. In D. Nehring, O. J. Madsen, E. Cabanas, C. Mills, & D. Kerrigan (Eds.), *Routledge international handbook of global therapeutic cultures*. Routledge.
Rivera, A. R., Gálvez-Mozo, A., & Tirado-Serrano, F. (2024). The imperative of happiness in positive psychology: Towards a psychopolitics of wellbeing. *New Ideas in Psychology, 72*, 101058. https://doi.org/10.1016/j.newideapsych.2023.101058
Roberts, I. (2007). How the obesity epidemic is aggravating global warming. *The New Scientist*. https://www.newscientist.com/article/mg19426105–600-how-the-obesity-epidemic-is-aggravating-global-warming/
Roberts, P. (1998, March 1). The new food anxiety: Food shapes our identity and influences how we see the world. *Psychology Today*. https://www.psychologytoday.com/intl/articles/199803/the-new-food-anxiety
Robinson, E. (2017). Overweight but unseen: A review of the underestimation of weight status and a visual normalization theory. *Obesity Review, 18*(10), 1200–1209. https://doi.org/10.1111/obr.12570
Robinson, E., Haynes, A., Sutin, A. R., & Daly, M. (2017). Telling people they are overweight: Helpful, harmful or beside the point? *International Journal of Obesity, 41*(8), 1160–1161. https://doi.org/10.1038/ijo.2017.85
Robson, D. (2024, June 16). Self-care: Why looking after No 1 isn't always best for your wellbeing. *The Guardian*. https://www.theguardian.com/society/article/2024/jun/16/wellbeing-selfcare-other-care-psychology-social
Rodgers, R. F., Laveway, K., Campos, P., & de Carvalho, P. H. B. (2023). Body image as a global mental health concern. *Global Mental Health, 10*, e9. https://doi.org/10.1017/gmh.2023.2
Rodgers, R. F., Paxton, S. J., Wertheim, E. H., & Fuller-Tyszkiewicz, M. (2024). Better than average Bopo: Identifying which body positive social media content is most helpful for body image among women. *Body Image, 51*, 101773. https://doi.org/10.1016/j.bodyim.2024.101773

Rodgers, R. F., Wertheim, E. H., Paxton, S. J., Tylka, T. L., & Harriger, J. A. (2022). #Bopo: Enhancing body image through body positive social media – evidence to date and research directions. *Body Image*, *41*, 367–374. https://doi.org/10.1016/j.bodyim.2022.03.008

Roesch, S. C., & Weiner, B. (2001). A meta-analytic review of coping with illness: Do causal attributions matter? *Journal of Psychosomatic Research*, *50*(4), 205–219. https://doi.org/10.1016/s0022-3999(01)00188-x

Rogers, P. J., & Smit, H. J. (2020). Food craving and food "addiction": A critical review of the evidence from a biopsychosocial perspective. *Pharmacology Biochemistry and Behavior*, *66*(1), 3–14. https://doi.org/10.1016/s0091-3057(00)00197-0

Romeo, A. (2020). Classical theories and contemporary examples of a complex object. *Sociétés*, *147*(1), 85. https://doi.org/10.3917/soc.147.0085

Rooney, T., Sharpe, L., Todd, J., Richmond, B., & Colagiuri, B. (2023). The relationship between expectancy, anxiety, and the nocebo effect: A systematic review and meta-analysis with recommendations for future research. *Health Psychology Review*, *17*(4), 550–577. https://doi.org/10.1080/17437199.2022.2125894

Rosa, H. (2013). *Social acceleration: A new theory of modernity* (J. Trejo-Mathys, Trans.). Columbia University Press.

Rosa, H. (2018, July 9). The idea of resonance as a sociological concept. *Global Dialogue*. https://globaldialogue.isa-sociology.org/articles/the-idea-of-resonance-as-a-sociological-concept

Rosa, H. (2019). *Resonance: A sociology of our relationship to the world* (J. C. Wagner, Trans.). Polity Press.

Rosa, H. (2020). *The uncontrollability of the world*. Polity Press.

Rose, N. (1998). *Inventing our selves: Psychology, power, and personhood*. Cambridge University Press.

Rose, N. (2018). *Our psychiatric future*. Polity.

Rosenthal, L. (2016). Incorporating intersectionality into psychology: An opportunity to promote social justice and equity. *American Psychologist*, *71*(6), 474–485. https://doi.org/10.1037/a0040323

Rosman, L., Gehi, A., & Lampert, R. (2020). When smartwatches contribute to health anxiety in patients with atrial fibrillation. *Cardiovascular Digital Health Journal*, *1*(1), 9–10. https://doi.org/10.1016/j.cvdhj.2020.06.004

Rosman, L., Lampert, R., Zhuo, S., Li, Q., Varma, N., Burg, M., Gaffey, A. E., Armbruster, T., & Gehi, A. (2024). Wearable devices, health care use, and psychological well-being in patients with atrial fibrillation. *Journal of the American Heart Association*, *13*(15), e033750. https://doi.org/10.1161/JAHA.123.033750

Rosmarin, D. H., & Pirutinsky, S. (2024). Response to anxiety treatment before, during, and after the COVID-19 pandemic. *PLoS ONE*, *19*(3), e0296949. https://doi.org/10.1371/journal.pone.0296949

Roszkowska, A., Pawlicka, M., Mroczek, A., Bałabuszek, K., & Nieradko-Iwanicka, B. (2019). Non-celiac gluten sensitivity: A review. *Medicina (Kaunas)*, *55*(6), 222. https://doi.org/10.3390/medicina55060222

Rubino, F., Cummings, D. E., Eckel, R. H., Cohen, R. V., Wilding, J. P. H., Brown, W. A., Stanford, F. C., Batterham, R. L., Farooqi, I. S., Farpour-Lambert, N. J., le Roux, C. W., Sattar, N., Baur, L. A., Morrison, K. M., Misra, A., Kadowaki, T., Tham, K. W., Sumithran, P., Garvey, W. T., . . . Mingrone, G. (2025). Definition and diagnostic criteria of clinical obesity. *The Lancet Diabetes & Endocrinology*. Advance online publication. https://doi.org/10.1016/S2213-8587(24)00316-4

Ruiter, R. A., Kessels, L. T., Peters, G. J., & Kok, G. (2014). Sixty years of fear appeal research: Current state of the evidence. *International Journal of Psychology*, *49*(2), 63–70. https://doi.org/10.1002/ijop.12042

Ruiu, M. L. (2020). Mismanagement of COVID-19: Lessons learned from Italy. *Journal of Risk Research*, *23*(7–8), 1007–1020. https://doi.org/10.1080/13669877.2020.1758755

Russo, M. T. (2020). The human body as a problem in post-modern culture. *Church, Communication and Culture*, *5*(1), 74–91. https://doi.org/10.1080/23753234.2020.1713010

Ryan, J., Edney, S., & Maher, C. (2019). Anxious or empowered? A cross-sectional study exploring how wearable activity trackers make their owners feel. *BMC Psychology*, *7*, 42. https://doi.org/10.1186/s40359-019-0315-y

Ryff, C. D. (1989). Happiness is everything, or is it? Explorations on the meaning of psychological well-being. *Journal of Personality and Social Psychology*, *57*(6), 1069–1081. https://doi.org/10.1037/0022-3514.57.6.1069

Saguy, A. C., & Almeling, R. (2008). Fat in the fire? Science, the news media, and the "obesity epidemic." *Sociology Forum*, *23*, 53–83. https://doi.org/10.1111/j.1600-0838.2004.00399.x-i1

Sale&Pepe Editorial Team. (n.d.). Gluten free: For health or for fashion? *Sale & Pepe*. https://www.salepepe.com/senza-glutine-salute-moda

Sallay, V., Martos, T., Lucza, L., Weiland, A., Stegers-Jager, K. M., Vermeir, P., Mariman, A. N. M., & Csabai, M. (2022). Medical educators' experiences on medically unexplained symptoms and intercultural communication: An expert focus group study. *BMC Medical Education*, *22*, 310. https://doi.org/10.1186/s12909-022-03275-0

Salles, A. (2021). Can 'big' be healthy? Yes – and no. *Medscape*. https://www.medscape.com/viewarticle/944165

Sallin, K., Evers, K., Jarbin, H., Joelsson, L., & Petrovic, P. (2023). Separation and not residency permit restores function in resignation syndrome: A retrospective cohort study. *European Child and Adolescent Psychiatry*, *32*(1), 75–86. https://doi.org/10.1007/s00787-021-01833-3

Sallin, K., Lagercrantz, H., Evers, K., Engström, I., Hjern, A., & Petrovic, P. (2016). Resignation syndrome: Catatonia? Culture-bound? *Frontiers in Behavioral Neuroscience*, *10*, 7. https://doi.org/10.3389/fnbeh.2016.00007

Samuelson, K. (Director), & Haptas, J. (Director). (2019). *Life overtakes me* [Film]. Netflix.

Santomauro, D. F., Whieford, H. A., & Ferrari, A. J. (2021). Global prevalence and burden of depressive and anxiety disorders in 204 countries and territories in 2020 due to the COVID-19 pandemic. *The Lancet*, *398*(10312), 1700–1712. https://doi.org/10.1016/s0140-6736(21)02800–2

Sauvayre, R. (2021). Ethics of belief, trust, and epistemic value: The case of the scientific controversy surrounding the measles vaccine. *Journal of Leadership Accountability and Ethics*, *18*(4), 24–34.

Schaumburg, H. H., Byck, R., Gerstl, R., & Mashman, J. H. (1969). Monosodium L-glutamate: Its pharmacology and role in the Chinese restaurant syndrome. *Science*, *163*, 826–828. https://doi.org/10.1126/science.163.3869.826

Scheier, M. F., Wrosch, C., Baum, A., Cohen, S., Martire, L. M., Matthews, K. A., Schulz, R., & Zdaniuk, B. (2006). The life engagement test: Assessing purpose in life. *Journal of Behavioral Medicine*, *29*(3), 291–298. https://doi.org/10.1007/s10865-005-9044-1

Schimmenti, A. (2023). Beyond addiction: Rethinking problematic internet use from a motivational framework. *Clinical Neuropsychiatry*, *20*(6), 471–478. https://doi.org/10.36131/cnfioritieditore20230601

Schnell, T. (2009). The sources of meaning and meaning in life questionnaire: Relations to demographics and well-being. *The Journal of Positive Psychology*, *4*(6), 483–499. https://doi.org/10.1080/17439760903271074

Schnell, T., & Krampe, H. (2022). Meaningfulness protects from and crisis of meaning exacerbates general mental distress longitudinally. *BMC Psychiatry*, *22*(1), 1–9. https://doi.org/10.1186/s12888-022-03921-3

Schnittker, J. (2021). *Unnerved: Anxiety, social change, and the transformation of modern mental health*. Columbia University Press.

Schultchen, D., Terhorst, Y., Holderied, T., Stach, M., Messner, E. M., Baumeister, H., & Sander, L. B. (2021). Stay present with your phone: A systematic review and standardized rating of mindfulness apps in European app stores. *International Journal of Behavioral Medicine*, *28*(5), 552–560. https://doi.org/10.1007/s12529-020-09944-y

Schulz, P. J., & Nakamoto, K. (2022). The perils of misinformation: When health literacy goes awry. *Nature Reviews Nephrology*, *18*(3), 135–136. https://doi.org/10.1038/s41581-021-00534-z

Schwartz, A. (2018, January 8). Improving ourselves to death: What the self-help gurus and their critics reveal about our times. *The New Yorker*. https://www.newyorker.com/magazine/2018/01/15/improving-ourselves-to-death

Schweitzer, A. M., Dišković, A., Krongauz, V., Newman, J., Tomažič, J., & Yancheva, N. (2023). Addressing HIV stigma in healthcare, community, and legislative settings in Central and Eastern Europe. *AIDS Research and Therapy*, *20*, 87. https://doi.org/10.1186/s12981-023-00585-1

Seligman, M. E. (1975). *Helplessness: On depression, development, and death*. W. H. Freeman.

Sergi, C., Villanacci, V., & Carroccio, A. (2021). Non-celiac wheat sensitivity: Rationality and irrationality of a gluten-free diet in individuals affected with non-celiac disease: A review. *BMC Gastroenterology*, *21*(5). https://doi.org/10.1186/s12876-020-01568-6

Seto, H., & Nakao, M. (2017). Relationships between catastrophic thought, bodily sensations and physical symptoms. *BioPsychoSocial Medicine*, *11*, 28. https://doi.org/10.1186/s13030-017-0110-z

Sewaybricker, L. E., & Massola, G. M. (2023). Against well-being: A critique of positive psychology. *History of the Human Sciences*, *36*(1), 131–148. https://doi.org/10.1177/09526951221114733

Shah, Y. B., Glatter, R., & Madad, S. (2022). In layman's terms: The power and problem of science communication. *Disaster Medicine and Public Health Preparedness*, *16*(6), 2245–2247. https://doi.org/10.1017/dmp.2022.131

Sham, S., Shiwlani, S., Kirshan Kumar, S., Bai, P., & Bendari, A. (2024). Empowering patients through digital health literacy and access to electronic medical records (EMRs) in the developing world. *Cureus*, *16*(4), e57527. https://doi.org/10.7759/cureus.57527

Sharon, T. (2017). Self-tracking for health and the quantified self: Re-articulating autonomy, solidarity, and authenticity in an age of personalized healthcare. *Philosophy & Technology*, *30*, 93–121. https://doi.org/10.1007/s13347-016-0215-5

Sharp, G., Bilal, M., Fernando, A. N., & de Boer, K. (2023). Examining health professional perspectives on social media body image movements: A qualitative exploration. *Body Image*, *46*, 230–237. https://doi.org/10.1016/j.bodyim.2023.06.004

Shetty, S. A., Chandini, S., Fernandes, S. L., & Safeekh, A. T. (2020). Hysteria: A historical perspective. *Archives of Medicine and Health Sciences*, *8*(2), 312–315. https://doi.org/10.4103/amhs.amhs_220_20

Shewale, R. (2024, March 24). Smartwatch statistics 2024: Worldwide market data. *Demandsage*. https://www.demandsage.com/smartwatch-statistics/

Shi, R., Liu, Q., & Wu, G. (2023). Risk perception and sense of public health safety: The mediating role of emotional perception. *Sustainability*, *15*(21), 15632. https://doi.org/10.3390/su152115632

Shi, Z., Du, X., Li, J., Hou, R., Sun, J., & Marohabutr, T. (2024). Factors influencing digital health literacy among older adults: A scoping review. *Frontiers in Public Health*, *12*, 1447747. https://doi.org/10.3389/fpubh.2024.1447747

Simons, G., & Baldwin, D. S. (2021). A critical review of the definition of 'wellbeing' for doctors and their patients in a post-COVID-19 era. *International Journal of Social Psychiatry*, *67*(8), 984–991. https://doi.org/10.1177/00207640211032259

Single Care Team. (2022). Anxiety statistics 2022. *SingleCare*. https://www.singlecare.com

Slovic, P. (2010). *The feeling of risk: New perspectives on risk perception*. Routledge.

Smith, D. (2012a, January 14). It's still the 'age of anxiety.' Or is it? *The New York Times.* https://archive.nytimes.com/opinionator.blogs.nytimes.com/2012/01/14/its-still-the-age-of-anxiety-or-is-it/

Smith, D. (2012b). *Monkey mind: A memoir of anxiety.* Simon & Schuster.

Snelling, P. C. (2015). Who can blame who for what and how in responsibility for health? *Nursing Philosophy, 16,* 3–18. https://doi.org/10.1111/nup.12061

Sobczak, C. (2014). *Embody: A guide to celebrating your unique body (and quieting that critical voice!).* Gürze Books.

Sorid, S. D., Yap, D. L., Bravo, A. J., & Behar, E. (2023). The moderating role of intolerance of uncertainty in the relationship between health anxiety and pandemic-related stress. *Cognitive Therapy and Research, 47*(3), 340–349. https://doi.org/10.1007/s10608-023-10365-w

Spadine, M., & Patterson, M. S. (2022). Social influence on fad diet use: A systematic literature review. *Nutrition and Health, 28*(3), 369–388. https://doi.org/10.1177/02601060211072370.

Sperber, A. D., Bangdiwala, S. I., Drossman, D. A., Ghoshal, U. C., Simrén, M., Tack, J., Whitehead, W. E., Dumitrascu, D. L., Fang, X., Fukudo, S., Kellow, J., Okeke, E., Quigley, E. M. M., Schmulson, M., Whorwell, P., Archampong, T., Adibi, P., Andresen, V., Benninga, M. A., . . . Palsson, O. S. (2021). Worldwide prevalence and burden of functional gastrointestinal disorders: Results of the Rome Foundation global study. *Gastroenterology, 160*(1), 99–114.e3. https://doi.org/10.1053/j.gastro.2020.04.014

Splevins, K., Cohen, K., Bowley, J., & Joseph, S. (2010). Theories of posttraumatic growth: Cross-cultural perspectives. *Journal of Loss and Trauma, 15*(3), 259–277. https://doi.org/10.1080/15325020903382111

Stamp, N. (2019). Berating Nike for plus-size mannequins is no war on obesity – it's just war on bigger bodies. *The Guardian.* https://www.theguardian.com/commentisfree/2019/jun/12/berating-nike-for-plus-size-mannequins-is-no-war-on-obesity-its-just-war-on-bigger-bodies

Starcevic, V. (2017). Cyberchondria: Challenges of problematic online searches for health-related information. *Psychotherapy and Psychosomatics, 86*(3), 129–133. https://doi.org/10.1159/000465525

Starcevic, V. (2020). Problematic and compulsive online health research: The two faces of cyberchondria. *Clinical Psychology: Science and Practice, 27*(2), e12320. https://doi.org/10.1111/cpsp.12320

Starcevic, V. (2023). Keeping Dr. Google under control: How to prevent and manage cyberchondria. *World Psychiatry, 22*(2), 233–234. https://doi.org/10.1002/wps.21076

Starcevic, V., & Berle, D. (2015). Cyberchondria: An old phenomenon in a new guise? In E. Aboujaoude & V. Starcevic (Eds.), *Mental health in the digital age: Grave dangers, great promise* (pp. 106–117). Oxford University Press.

Starcevic, V., & Noyes, R., Jr. (Eds.). (2014). *Hypochondriasis and health anxiety: A guide for clinicians.* Oxford University Press.

Starcevic, V., Schimmenti, A., Billieux, J., & Berle, D. (2020). Cyberchondria in the time of the COVID-19 pandemic. *Human Behavior and Emerging Technologies, 3*(1), 53–62. https://doi.org/10.1002/hbe2.233

Staszak, J.-F. (2009). Other/otherness. In *International encyclopedia of human geography: A 12-volume set* (Eds. Kitchin & Thrift). Elsevier Science.

Statista Research Department. (2024, July 22). Number of users of smartwatches worldwide from 2020 to 2029. *Statista.* https://www.statista.com/forecasts/1314339/worldwide-users-of-smartwatches

Steel, P., Taras, V., Uggerslev, K., & Bosco, F. (2018). The happy culture: A theoretical, meta-analytic, and empirical review of the relationship between culture, wealth, and subjective well-being. *Personality and Social Psychology Review, 22*(2), 128–169. https://doi.org/10.1177/1088868317721372

Steger, M. F. (2024). Regenerative positive psychology: A call to reorient wellbeing science to meet the realities of our world. *The Journal of Positive Psychology*. https://doi.org/10.1080/17439760.2024.2365259

Steiger, A. E., Fend, H. A., & Allemand, M. (2015). Testing the vulnerability and scar models of self-esteem and depressive symptoms from adolescence to middle adulthood and across generations. *Developmental Psychology*, *51*(2), 236–247. https://doi.org/10.1037/a0038478

Stephens, G. (2014). Insights on the gluten-free market: Once believed to be a passing fad, the gluten-free foods category has evolved to become a mainstream star. *Nutraceuticals World*, *17*(9), 24–26. https://www.nutraceuticalsworld.com/issues/2014-11/view_columns/insights-on-the-gluten-free-market/

Stone, L. (2014). Blame, shame and hopelessness: Medically unexplained symptoms and the 'heartsink' experience. *Australian Family Physician*, *43*(4), 191–195.

Stossel, S. (2014). *My age of anxiety: Fear, hope, dread, and the search for peace of mind*. Vintage.

Stoumpos, A. I., Kitsios, F., & Talias, M. A. (2023). Digital transformation in healthcare: Technology acceptance and its applications. *International Journal of Environmental Research and Public Health*, *20*(4), 3407. https://doi.org/10.3390/ijerph20043407

Strahler, J. (2019). Sex differences in orthorexic eating behaviors: A systematic review and meta-analytical integration. *Nutrition*, *67–68*, 110534. https://doi.org/10.1016/j.nut.2019.06.015

Straker, G., & Winship, J. (2023, October 29). Health anxiety can be all-consuming. Accepting uncertainty is an important step. *The Guardian*. https://www.theguardian.com/commentisfree/2023/oct/29/health-anxiety-can-be-all-consuming-accepting-uncertainty-is-an-important-step

Suslovic, B., & Lett, E. (2024). Resilience is an adverse event: A critical discussion of resilience theory in health services research and public health. *Community Health Equity Research & Policy*, *44*(3), 339–343. https://doi.org/10.1177/2752535X231159721

Sutin, A. R., Stephan, Y., & Terracciano, A. (2015). Weight discrimination and risk of mortality. *Psychological Science*, *26*(11), 1803–1811. https://doi.org/10.1177/0956797615601103

Swami, V., Weis, L., Barron, D., & Furnham, A. (2018). Positive body image is positively associated with hedonic (emotional) and eudaimonic (psychological and social) well-being in British adults. *The Journal of Social Psychology*, *158*(5), 541–552. https://doi.org/10.1080/00224545.2017.1392278

Swift, J. A., Hanlon, S., El-Redy, L., Puhl, R. M., & Glazebrook, C. (2013). Weight bias among UK trainee dietitians, doctors, nurses and nutritionists. *Journal of Human Nutrition and Dietetics*, *26*(4), 395–402. https://doi.org/10.1111/jhn.12019

Szűcs, V., Fazakas, Z., Farr, A. M., & Tarcea, M. (2019). Quality of life of consumers following a gluten-free diet: Results of a questionnaire survey in Hungary and Romania. *Orvosi Hetilap*, *160*(25), 980–986. https://doi.org/10.1556/650.2019.31421

Taebi, M., Kariman, N., Montazeri, A., & Alavi Majd, H. (2021). Infertility stigma: A qualitative study on feelings and experiences of infertile women. *International Journal of Fertility & Sterility*, *15*(3), 189–196. https://doi.org/10.22074/IJFS.2021.139093.1039

Takeda, A. (2017, May 23). 16 famous men who have had prostate cancer. *Everyday Health*. https://www.everydayhealth.com

Talumaa, B., Brown, A., Batterham, R. L., & Kalea, A. Z. (2022). Effective strategies in ending weight stigma in healthcare. *Obesity Reviews*, *23*(10), e13494. https://doi.org/10.1111/obr.13494

Tanemura, N., Kakizaki, M., Kusumi, T., Onodera, R., & Chiba, T. (2022). Levels of trust in risk-only negative health messages issued by public agencies: A quantitative research-based mindsponge framework. *Humanities and Social Sciences Communications*, *9*, 388. https://doi.org/10.1057/s41599-022-01415-x

Tangney, J. P., Stuewig, J., & Mashek, D. J. (2007). Moral emotions and moral behavior. *Annual Review of Psychology, 58*, 345–372. https://doi.org/10.1146/annurev.psych.56.091103.070145

Taylor, H. (2010). *Cyberchondriacs on the rise? Those who go online for healthcare information continues to increase*. http://www.harrisinteractive.com/vault/HI-Harris-Poll-Cyberchondriacs-2010-08-04.pdf

Tedeschi, R., Moore, B. A., Falke, K., & Goldberg, J. (2020). *Transformed by trauma: Stories of posttraumatic growth*. Independently published.

Tedeschi, R., Shakespeare-Finch, J., & Taku, K. (2018). *Posttraumatic growth: Theory, research, and applications*. Routledge.

Tedeschi, R. G., & Calhoun, L. G. (1996). The posttraumatic growth inventory: Measuring the positive legacy of trauma. *Journal of Traumatic Stress, 9*(3), 455–471. https://doi.org/10.1007/BF02103658

Tedeschi, R. G., & Calhoun, L. G. (2004). Posttraumatic growth: Conceptual foundations and empirical evidence. *Psychological Inquiry, 15*(1), 1–18. https://doi.org/10.1207/s15327965pli1501_01

Teepe, G. W., Glase, E. M., & Reips, U. D. (2023). Increasing digitalization is associated with anxiety and depression: A Google Ngram analysis. *PLoS ONE, 18*(4), e0284091. https://doi.org/10.1371/journal.pone.0284091

Thomas, J. D. L. (2012). When patients seem overly optimistic. *Virtual Mentor, 14*(7), 539–544. https://doi.org/10.1001/virtualmentor.2012.14.7.ecas2-1207

Thomas, S. P. (2017). Resignation syndrome: Is it a new phenomenon or is it catatonia? *Issues in Mental Health Nursing, 38*(7), 531–532. https://doi.org/10.1080/01612840.2017.1341229

Thomas, S. P. (2023). Addressing gaps in knowledge about cyberchondria. *Issues in Mental Health Nursing, 44*(7), 583–584. https://doi.org/10.1080/01612840.2023.2229718

Thomas, T. W., & Cankurt, M. (2024). Influence of food environments on dietary habits: Insights from a quasi-experimental research. *Foods, 13*(13), 2013. https://doi.org/10.3390/foods13132013

Thorgaard, M. V. (2017). Health anxiety and illness behavior in children of mothers with severe health anxiety. *Danish Medical Journal, 64*(5), B5365.

Thorgaard, M. V., Frostholm, L., & Rask, C. U. (2018). Childhood and family factors in the development of health anxiety: A systematic review. *Children's Health Care, 47*(2), 198–238. https://doi.org/10.1080/02739615.2017.1318390

Tidy, J. (2024, January 5). Character.ai: Young people turning to AI therapist bots. *BBC News*. https://www.bbc.com/news/technology-67872693

Tiggemann, M. (2024). A few reflections on positive body image and body neutrality (aided by Tom Cash's model). *Body Image, 51*, 101790. https://doi.org/10.1016/j.bodyim.2024.101790

Tiggemann, M., & McGill, B. (2004). The role of social comparison in the effect of magazine advertisements on women's mood and body dissatisfaction. *Journal of Social and Clinical Psychology, 23*(1), 23–44. https://doi.org/10.1521/jscp.23.1.23.26991

Tone, A. (2017). *The age of anxiety: A history of America's turbulent affair with tranquilizers*. GF Books, Inc.

Topol, E. (2013). *The creative destruction of medicine: How the digital revolution will create better health care*. Basic Books.

Tort-Nasarre, G., Pollina-Pocallet, M., Ferrer Suquet, Y., Ortega Bravo, M., Vilafranca Cartagena, M., & Artigues-Barberà, E. (2023). Positive body image: A qualitative study on the successful experiences of adolescents, teachers, and parents. *International Journal of Qualitative Studies on Health and Well-Being, 18*(1). https://doi.org/10.1080/17482631.2023.2170007

Townshed, P. (2019). *The age of anxiety: A novel*. Hachette Books.

Travers, M. (2022, November 13). A psychologist tells you why you need to escape the toxic world of self-help. *Forbes*. https://www.forbes.com/sites/traversmark/2022/11/13/a-psychologist-tells-you-why-you-need-to-escape-the-toxic-world-of-self-help/

Treufeldt, H., & Burton, C. (2024). Stigmatisation in medical encounters for persistent physical symptoms/functional disorders: Scoping review and thematic synthesis. *Patient Education and Counseling, 123*, 108198. https://doi.org/10.1016/j.pec.2024.108198

Trujillo, C. A. (2018). The complementary role of affect-based and cognitive heuristics to make decisions under conditions of ambivalence and complexity. *PLoS ONE, 13*(11), e0206724. https://doi.org/10.1371/journal.pone.0206724

Tsawaab, A. H. (2023). The impact of body positivity in fashion advertising on customer perceptions and purchase intentions. *International Journal of Multidisciplinary Business and Education Research, 4*(8), 2769–2784. https://doi.org/10.11594/ijmaber.04.08.10

Turkle, S. (2024, March). *Who do we become when we talk to machines? An MIT exploration of generative AI.* https://doi.org/10.21428/e4baedd9.caa10d84

Turner, P. G., & Lefevre, C. E. (2017). Instagram use is linked to increased symptoms of orthorexia nervosa. *Eating and Weight Disorders, 22*(2), 277–284. https://doi.org/10.1007/s40519-017-0364-2

Twenge, J. M. (2000). The age of anxiety? The birth cohort change in anxiety and neuroticism, 1952–1993. *Journal of Personality and Social Psychology, 79*(6), 1007–1021. https://doi.org/10.1037/0022-3514.79.6.1007

Twenge, J. M., & Campbell, W. K. (2009). *The narcissism epidemic: Living in the age of entitlement.* Free Press.

Tylka, T. L. (2011). Positive psychology perspectives on body image. In T. F. Cash & L. Smolak (Eds.), *Body image: A handbook of science, practice, and prevention* (pp. 56–64). Guilford Press.

Tylka, T. L., & Piran, N. (2019). The developmental theory of embodiment: Protective social factors that enhance positive embodiment. In T. L. Tylka (Ed.), *Handbook of positive body image and embodiment: Constructs, protective factors, and interventions* (pp. 56–64). Oxford Academic.

Tylka, T. L., & Wood-Barcalow, N. L. (2015). What is and what is not positive body image? Conceptual foundations and construct definition. *Body Image, 14*, 118–129. https://doi.org/10.1016/j.bodyim.2015.04.001

Tyrer, P., Cooper, S., Tyrer, H., Wang, D., & Bassett, P. (2019). Increase in the prevalence of health anxiety in medical clinics: Possible cyberchondria. *International Journal of Social Psychiatry, 65*(7–8), 566–569. https://doi.org/10.1177/0020764019866231

Umberson, D., Donnelly, R., & Pollitt, A. M. (2018). Marriage, social control, and health behavior: A dyadic analysis of same-sex and different-sex couples. *Journal of Health and Social Behavior, 59*(3), 429–446. https://doi.org/10.1177/0022146518790560

UNICEF. (2022). *Climate heroes take action on World Children's Day.* UNICEF. https://www.unicef.org/sop/stories/climate-heroes-take-action-world-childrens-day

van Baal, K., Stiel, S., & Schulte, P. (2023). Public perceptions of climate change and health: A cross-sectional survey study. *International Journal of Environmental Research and Public Health, 20*(2), 1464. https://doi.org/10.3390/ijerph20021464

Van Dam, N. T., van Vugt, M. K., Vago, D. R., Schmalzl, L., Saron, C. D., Olendzki, A., Meissner, T., Lazar, S. W., Kerr, C. E., Gorchov, J., Fox, K. C. R., Field, B. A., Britton, W. B., Brefczynski-Lewis, J. A., & Meyer, D. E. (2018). Mind the hype: A critical evaluation and prescriptive agenda for research on mindfulness and meditation. *Perspectives on Psychological Science, 13*(1), 36–61. https://doi.org/10.1177/1745691617709589

Van den Heuvel, O. A., Veale, D., & Stein, D. J. (2014). Hypochondriasis: Considerations for ICD–11. *Brazilian Journal of Psychiatry, 36*(Suppl. 1), 21–27. https://doi.org/10.1590/1516-4446-2013-1218

van Dyke, C. (2018). Eat y'self fitter: Orthorexia, health, and gender. In A. Barnhill, M. Budolfson, & T. Doggett (Eds.), *Oxford handbook of food ethics* (pp. 553–571). Oxford University Press.

van Krieken, R. (2014). Norbert Elias and emotions in history. In D. Lemmings & A. Brooks (Eds.), *Emotions and social change: Historical and sociological perspectives* (pp. 19–42). Routledge.

van Zyl, L. E., Gaffaney, J., van der Vaart, L., Dik, B. J., & Donaldson, S. I. (2023). The critiques and criticisms of positive psychology: A systematic review. *The Journal of Positive Psychology*, *19*(2), 206–235. https://doi.org/10.1080/17439760.2023.2178956

Verlie, B. (2022). *Learning to live with climate change: From anxiety to transformation*. Routledge.

Vermeir, P., Mariman, A., Lucza, L., Sallay, V., Weiland, A., Stegers-Jager, K. M., & Vogelaers, D. (2021). Epidemiology and organization of care in medically unexplained symptoms: A systematic review with a focus on cultural diversity and migrants. *International Journal of Clinical Practice*, *75*(12), e14855. https://doi.org/10.1111/ijcp.14855

Villarroya, F., & Giralt, M. (2024). Faced with a double challenge: Obesity and climate change. *BMI Journal*. https://doi.org/10.53435/funj.00987

Vismara, M., Caricasole, V., Starcevic, V., Cinosi, E., Dell'Osso, B., Martinotti, G., & Fineberg, N. A. (2020). Is cyberchondria a new transdiagnostic digital compulsive syndrome? A systematic review of the evidence. *Comprehensive Psychiatry, 99*, 152167. https://doi.org/10.1016/j.comppsych.2020.152167

Vos, J. (2016). Working with meaning in life in mental health care: A systematic literature review of the practices and effectiveness of meaning-centred therapies. In P. Russo-Netzer, S. E. Schulenberg, & A. Batthyany (Eds.), *Clinical perspectives on meaning: Positive and existential psychotherapy* (pp. 59–89). Springer.

Voth, J., & Sirois, F. M. (2009). The role of self-blame and responsibility in adjustment to inflammatory bowel disease. *Rehabilitation Psychology*, *54*(1), 99–108. https://doi.org/10.1037/a0014739

Vudathaneni, V. K. P., Lanke, R. B., Mudaliyar, M. C., Movva, K. V., Kalluri, M., & Boyapati, R. (2024). The impact of telemedicine and remote patient monitoring on healthcare delivery: A comprehensive evaluation. *Cureus*, *16*(3), e55534. https://doi.org/10.7759/cureus.55534

Wagner, W. (2020). Social representation theory: An historical outline. *Oxford Research Encyclopedia of Psychology*. https://doi.org/10.1093/acrefore/9780190236557.001.0001/acrefore-9780190236557-e-606

Walsh, M. J., & Baker, S. A. (2020). Clean eating and Instagram: Purity, defilement, and the idealization of food. *Food, Culture & Society*. https://doi.org/10.1080/15528014.2020.1806636

Walsh, Z. (2016). A meta-critique of mindfulness critiques: From McMindfulness to critical mindfulness. In R. Purser, D. Forbes, & A. Burke (Eds.), *Handbook of mindfulness. Mindfulness in behavioral health* (pp. 231–250). Springer. https://doi.org/10.1007/978-3-319-44019-4_11

Wanger, J. (2024). Is technology creating an anxious generation? *World Economic Forum Annual Meeting*. https://www.weforum.org/stories/2024/10/technology-creating-an-anxious-generation/

Wardell, A. (2024, March 4). How hyper-individualistic self-care culture has lost its way. *Medium*. https://medium.com/@amber_wardell/how-hyper-individualistic-self-care-culture-has-lost-its-way-4b4b9a097b0d

Watson, D., Wallace, J., Land, C., & Patey, J. (2023). Re-organising wellbeing: Contexts, critiques, and contestations of dominant wellbeing narratives. *Organization*, *30*(3), 441–452. https://doi.org/10.1177/13505084231156267

Watson, S. (2023, October 20). Famous men who beat prostate cancer (or caught it just in time). *Health Central*. https://www.healthcentral.com

Western, S. (2012). The wounded self and celebrated self. In S. Western (Ed.), *Introduction to coaching and mentoring: A critical text*. Sage Academic Books. https://doi.org/10.4135/9781446251577.n1

White, R. W., & Horvitz, E. (2009a). Cyberchondria: Studies of the escalation of medical concerns in web search. *ACM Transactions on Information Systems*, *27*(4), 23. https://doi.org/10.1145/1629096.1629101
White, R. W., & Horvitz, E. (2009b). Experiences with web search on medical concerns and self-diagnosis. In *Proceedings from the American medical informatics association annual symposium* (pp. 696–700). Curran Associates.
Whitney, D., & Taku, K. (2023). Application of a theoretical model of posttraumatic growth to distinguish between posttraumatic growth and illusory growth. In R. Berger (Ed.), *The Routledge international handbook of posttraumatic growth*. https://doi.org/10.4324/9781032208688
Widiger, T. A., & Samuel, D. B. (2005). Diagnostic categories or dimensions? A question for the *Diagnostic and statistical manual of mental disorders – fifth edition*. *Journal of Abnormal Psychology*, *114*(4), 494–504. https://doi.org/10.1037/0021-843X.114.4.494
Wieczorek, M., O'Brolchain, F., Saghai, Y., & Gordijn, B. (2022). The ethics of self-tracking: A comprehensive review of the literature. *Ethics & Behavior*, *33*(4), 239–271. https://doi.org/10.1080/10508422.2022.2082969
Wilkinson, I. (2009). *Risk, vulnerability, and everyday life (The new sociology)*. Routledge.
Will, C. M., Henwood, F., Weiner, K., & Williams, R. (2020). Negotiating the practical ethics of 'self-tracking' in intimate relationships: Looking for care in healthy living. *Social Science & Medicine*, *266*, 113301. https://doi.org/10.1016/j.socscimed.2020.113301
Williams, A. (2014, September 19). The paleo lifestyle: The way, way, way back. *The New York Times*. https://www.nytimes.com/2014/09/21/fashion/the-paleo-lifestyle-the-way-way-way-back.html
Wissing, M. P. (2022). Beyond the "third wave of positive psychology": Challenges and opportunities for the future. *Frontiers in Psychology*, *12*. https://doi.org/10.3389/fpsyg.2021.795067
Wolf, G. (2009). Know thyself: Tracking every facet of life, from sleep to mood to pain, 24/7/365. *Wired*. https://www.wired.com/2009/06/lbnp-knowthyself/
Wolf, G. (2016). The quantified self: Reverse engineering. In D. Nafus (Ed.), *Quantified: Biosensing technologies in everyday life* (pp. 141–162). MIT Press. https://doi.org/10.7551/mitpress/10293.003.0007
Wong, K. P., Tse, M. M. Y., & Qin, J. (2022). Effectiveness of virtual reality-based interventions for managing chronic pain on pain reduction, anxiety, depression, and mood: A systematic review. *Healthcare*, *10*(10), 2047. https://doi.org/10.3390/healthcare10102047
Wong, P. T. (2011). Positive psychology 2.0: Towards a balanced interactive model of the good life. *Canadian Psychology/Psychologie Canadienne*, *52*(2), 69–81. https://doi.org/10.1037/a0022511
Woo, S., Zhou, W., & Larson, J. L. (2021). Stigma experiences in people with chronic obstructive pulmonary disease: An integrative review. *International Journal of Chronic Obstructive Pulmonary Disease*, *16*, 1647–1659. https://doi.org/10.2147/COPD.S306874
Wood, A. M., & Joseph, S. (2010). The absence of positive psychological (eudemonic) well-being as a risk factor for depression: A ten-year cohort study. *Journal of Affective Disorders*, *122*(3), 213–217. https://doi.org/10.1016/j.jad.2009.06.032
Wood-Barcalow, N. L., Alleva, J. M., & Tylka, T. L. (2024). Revisiting positive body image to demonstrate how body neutrality is not new. *Body Image*, *50*, 101741. https://doi.org/10.1016/j.bodyim.2024.101741
Wood-Barcalow, N. L., Tylka, T. L., & Augustus-Horvath, C. L. (2010). "But I like my body": Positive body image characteristics and a holistic model for young-adult women. *Body Image*, *7*(2), 106–116. https://doi.org/10.1016/j.bodyim.2010.01.001
World Health Organization (2019). *International statistical classification of diseases and related health problems* (11th ed.). https://icd.who.int/

Wróblewska, B., Szyc, A. M., Markiewicz, L. H., Zakrzewska, M., & Romaszko, E. (2018). Increased prevalence of eating disorders as a biopsychosocial implication of food allergy. *PLoS ONE, 13*(6), e0198607. https://doi.org/10.1371/journal.pone.0198607

Wu, J., Snell, G., & Samji, H. (2020). Climate anxiety in young people: A call to action. *The Lancet Planetary Health, 4*(10), e435–e436. https://doi.org/10.1016/S2542-5196(20)30223–0

Xiao, Y., Baes, N., Vylomova, E., & Haslam, N. (2023). Have the concepts of 'anxiety' and 'depression' been normalized or pathologized? A corpus study of historical semantic change. *PLoS ONE, 18*(6), e0288027. https://doi.org/10.1371/journal.pone.0288027

Xiong, Z., Zhang, L., Li, Z., Xu, W., Zhang, Y., & Ye, T. (2021). Frequency of online health information seeking and types of information sought among the general Chinese population: Cross-sectional study. *Journal of Medical Internet Research, 23*(12), e30855. https://doi.org/10.2196/30855

Yam, K. (2020, January 14). Eddie Huang on racial insensitivities behind MSG, Chinese food criticisms. *NBC News*. https://www.nbcnews.com/news/asian-america/eddie-huang-racial-insensitivities-behind-msg-chinese-food-criticisms-n1115386

Yerkes, R. M., & Dodson, J. D. (1908). The relation of strength of stimulus to rapidity of habit-formation. *Journal of Comparative Neurology and Psychology, 18*(1), 459–482.

Yeung, A., Norton, R., Dean, T., Nagaswami, M., Yeung, A., Vuky, C., Mischoulon, D., & Borba, C. (2021). Depressed Chinese Americans present predominantly psychological symptoms: A new trend or different outcomes due to methodological differences? *Asian Journal of Psychiatry, 61*, 102684. https://doi.org/10.1016/j.ajp.2021.102684

Younis, H. A., Eisa, T. A. E., Nasser, M., Sahib, T. M., Noor, A. A., Alyasiri, O. M., Salisu, S., Hayder, I. M., & Younis, H. A. (2024). A systematic review and meta-analysis of artificial intelligence tools in medicine and healthcare: Applications, considerations, limitations, motivation, and challenges. *Diagnostics, 14*(1), 109. https://doi.org/10.3390/diagnostics14010109

Yuen, E., Winter, N., Savira, F., Huggins, C. E., Nguyen, L., Cooper, P., Peeters, A., Anderson, K., Bhoyroo, R., Crowe, S., & Ugalde, A. (2024). Digital health literacy and its association with sociodemographic characteristics, health resource use, and health outcomes: Rapid review. *Interactive Journal of Medical Research, 13*, e46888. https://doi.org/10.2196/46888

Zanfirescu, A., Ungurianu, A., Tsatsakis, A. M., Nițulescu, G. M., Kouretas, D., Veskoukis, A., Tsoukalas, D., Engin, A. B., Aschner, M., & Margină, D. (2019). A review of the alleged health hazards of monosodium glutamate. *Comprehensive Reviews in Food Science and Food Safety, 18*(4), 1111–1134. https://doi.org/10.1111/1541-4337.12448

Zeller, B. (2015). Totem and taboo in the grocery store: Quasi-religious foodways in North America. *Scripta Instituti Donneriani Aboensis, 26*, 11–31. https://doi.org/10.30674/scripta.67444

Zeng, J., Yuan, M., & Huang, G. (2022). Individual characteristics or cultures? Public risk perception in the coronavirus pandemic. *Journal of Risk Research, 25*(11–12), 1413–1443. https://doi.org/10.1080/13669877.2022.2142951

Zerbini, C., De Canio, F., Martinelli, E., & Luceri, B. (2024). Are gluten-free products healthy for non-celiac consumers? How the perception of well-being moderates gluten-free addiction. *Food Quality and Preference, 118*(3), 105183. https://doi.org/10.1016/j.foodqual.2024.105183

Žižek, S. (2002). *Welcome to the desert of the real*. Verso.

INDEX

For Product Safety Concerns and Information please contact our
EU representative GPSR@taylorandfrancis.com Taylor & Francis
Verlag GmbH, Kaufingerstraße 24, 80331 München, Germany